CARING FOR PATIENTS, CARING FOR STUDENT NURSES

For a dear friend and colleague, Blair Collister

Caring for Patients, Caring for Student Nurses

ANNETTE M. JINKS

Routledge
Taylor & Francis Group
LONDON AND NEW YORK

First published 1997 by Ashgate Publishing

Reissued 2018 by Routledge
2 Park Square, Milton Park, Abingdon, Oxon OX14 4RN
605 Third Avenue, New York, NY 10017

Routledge is an imprint of the Taylor & Francis Group, an informa business

A Library of Congress record exists under LC control number: 97071716

ISBN 13: 978-1-138-61226-6 (hbk)
ISBN 13: 978-0-429-45961-0 (ebk)

Contents

Figures and tables

Acknowledgements

I am especially grateful to Professor Nick Boreham, for all his help and guidance. I also wish to thank Professor Christine Webb for her diligent proof reading and above all in making the publication of this book possible. I would also like to thank all my nurse teacher and student nurse colleagues who participated in this study and gave their time so generously. Finally my deepest and sincerest thanks to my husband for his unwavering support and understanding whilst I have been writing this book.

1 Introduction

The subject of this book is a study which examines the interrelationships between student–centred teaching and learning and patient–centred nursing care. The focal area of interest is if student nurses are taught using the principles of student–centred learning theories will these behaviours be replicated by students in their attitudes to the delivery of nursing care. Student–centred learning and teaching is defined as a cognitive theory of learning which has self–directed, experiential and problem–solving learning as key features. In nurse education the application of student–centred learning and teaching methods is shown to have been influenced by andragogical tenets. Patient–centred care is defined as nursing care delivered through use of the nursing process.

The study is conducted during a time of radical change in nurse education in Great Britain. For example, the advent of Project 2000 and changes to post–registration training have inherent aims to produce nurses who are 'knowledgeable doers' (United Kingdom Central Council 1986). An implicit purpose of these reforms in nurse education is to raise the quality of professional nursing care (Chandler 1991). Much interest has centred on learning and teaching philosophies and methodologies which will assist in achieving these aims (D'A Slevin and Lavery 1991). The English National Board (1989) also state that educational processes should be directed towards students being encouraged to 'take personal responsibility for their learning' and 'developing their intellectual abilities, self–awareness and self–direction'. Attention has therefore focused on student–centred learning as a means of delivering nurse education programmes which have the aim of improving the quality of professional nursing care.

Improving the quality of nursing care through the delivery of effective nurse education programmes is central to the debate regarding the theory:practice divide in nurse education (Hawkett 1989, Jarvis 1992a, McCaugherty 1991b). For example, endeavours to design nurse education programmes which marry with the realities of clinical practice, and produce nurses who are able to deliver effective nursing care are central aims of all nursing curricula. This study examines one area of this broad topic.

The nature of the research described in this book is attitude analysis. That is analysis of the attitudes of senior educational managers, nurse teachers and pre–registration student nurses with regard to student–centred learning and teaching and patient–centred nursing care. Radford and Govier (1980) state that in analysing attitudes a distinction is usually made between three components: cognitive, affective and behavioural. The cognitive component consists of beliefs or ideas which a person holds towards an attitude issue, the affective component being the feelings or emotional reactions which an individual displays towards an attitude issue, and the behavioural component the tendency or disposition to react in certain ways to an attitude issue.

In the study the first two components identified by Radford and Govier (1980) are of central interest. That is the beliefs and feelings the sample groups hold with regard to student–centredness and patient–centredness. The latter component, or the study of actual behaviours regarding student–centredness and patient–centredness, are not addressed in the present study. Therefore the findings are used to illustrate beliefs and feeling regarding the attitude issues at a given point in time. There is no attempt made to examine the consistency between espoused beliefs and feelings and actual behaviours due to the need to keep the present study within manageable limits. For example, classroom observations have not been undertaken to establish articulation of student–centred principles in nurse teacher/student nurse teaching and learning interactions. Neither have clinical observations been conducted to verify the extent of patient–centred philosophy is evident in student nurses' care delivery. The findings of the study therefore, cannot be used to establish current behaviours or to predict future behaviour. It is, however, recommended in the conclusions of this book that these areas are subject areas for future research.

With these limitations acknowledged it is, however, clear that inferences can be made between ideas and beliefs and actual behaviours regarding attitude issues. Therefore any consensus picture which may emerge pertaining to ideas and beliefs of either student–centredness or patient–centredness would give some indication of how teachers and student nurses may act in teaching, learning or nursing care situations.

The general consensus picture which emerges from the findings of the study is that care and care giving are identified as being of key importance in analysis of attitudes towards student–centredness and patient–centredness. Care is, however, defined not merely as cherishing or nurturing behaviours but in the context of the theoretical concepts pertaining to student–centred learning and teaching and patient–centred nursing care. Effective teaching behaviours through application of the ideas and beliefs inherent in concepts of individualism, humanism and empowerment are identified as underpinning the definitions of care used in the study, whether this be care for students or care for patients.

A national survey approach is taken in the study. Initial investigations are directed at establishing senior educational managers or 'official' attitudes towards student–centredness. At later points in the study the attitudes of nurse teachers and pre–registration student nurses are examined towards both student–centredness and patient–centredness. Data triangulation is the central feature of the research design. The aim being to achieve convergent validity with regard to the research findings. An investigation, at a national level, which examines the attitudes of senior educational managers, nurse teachers and pre–registration student nurses with regard to student–

centredness and its relationship to patient–centredness is therefore the focus of the study.

Initially, however, the research began with an interest to if student nurses are taught in a student–centred fashion by nurse teachers will this behaviour be replicated in nursing care settings. A review of literature review was subsequently conducted using student–centredness and patient–centredness as focal areas of investigation. The first part of the review is given in the following chapter, and relates to student–centred teaching and learning theories and how these theories are articulated in nurse education.

2 Theories of learning and teaching

This chapter is directed towards examining and evaluating the literature pertaining to student-centred learning, its philosophies and methodologies, and exploring how student-centred learning can be seen to improve the quality of professional nursing care in the context of patient-centred care.

Definitions of student-centred learning and teaching

Woods and Barrow (1985) state that the term 'person'.or 'pupil-centredness' is open to widely differing interpretations. Beckett and Wall (1985) and Nielsen (1992) describe how the term grew out the propositions of Rogers (1969), who placed emphasis on processes of learning and dismissed 'teaching as a vastly over-rated function'. Inherent in Rogers' beliefs are that independence in the process of seeking information is a more stable base for education than of transmitting static knowledge. The underpinning assumption in the latter is what is taught is learnt. Rogers' therefore advocated a move away from lecture methods towards active student participation in teaching and learning processes.

Rogers' (1969) position can, however, be related to a broader debate in the arena of educational philosophy. For example, the concept of learner-centredness can be seen to stem out of beliefs about how learning occurs.

Learning theories

Child (1986) identifies two major perspectives of learning theory, those of the behaviourists and cognitivists. These broad conceptualizations can be seen to arise from differences in philosophical views about the way human beings learn. For example, behaviourist theory is chiefly concerned with externally observable input and output, a stimulus and response theory. Cognitive theory, however, is based on beliefs that inner functions of human beings affect human behaviour and therefore learning. Examples of these inner functions include the part motivational and perceptual factors play in teaching and learning.

A central debate in the arena of nursing education relates to which learning theory should have primacy. Byrnes (1986), Carter (1979), Darbyshire (1991), Duffy (1986), Gott (1982), McKenzie (1985) and Mutzebaugh and Dunn (1976) describe the application of these theories of learning to teaching nursing. Explicit advocacy of a cognitivist approach in nursings' national statutory bodies in the United Kingdom may be demonstrated in the quotation given in the introduction to this book (ENB 1989). For example, the quotation gives promoting personal responsibility and self-direction as key aims of nurse education processes. Development of both of these qualities are associated with cognitive learning theories. Carter (1979), Darbyshire (1991), and McKenzie (1985) may be given as further examples of advocates of a cognitivist approach to teaching and learning in nurse education programmes.

Some authors, however, see an implicit adherence to behaviourist-type beliefs by nursings' statutory bodies in Great Britain. For example, Farmer (1992) sees Project 2000 proposals as predominantly following behaviourist training models of education. Similarly Rolfe (1993a) identifies that the transition to higher education ushered in by Project 2000 has signalled a return to traditional teaching methods in nurse education. Ashworth and Morrison (1991) give similar criticisms of the identification of registered nursing competences in the 1989 Nurses, Midwives and Health Visitors Act.

Application of behaviourist theory is also seen by some as appropriate in certain discrete areas of nurse education. Gott (1982), Mutzebaugh and Dunn (1976), and Stotts (1982) give examples of how behaviourist theory may be of relevance for skills training. Beattie (1987) gives a four-fold model of curriculum and identifies that the application of behaviourist theory as being appropriate to teaching and learning practical skills. Sturmey (1988) also describes how a behaviourist approach is pertinent to nursing those with learning disabilities. Sturmey concludes that more compliance by carers is achieved when behavioural objectives are used in care planning.

It is therefore seen that there is still controversy in nursing education surrounding the behaviourist/cognitivist dichotomy, and frequently an eclectic approach is still evident in respect of broader issues of nursing education theory.

Learner-centredness, however, can be seen to relate directly to Bruner's (1966) theory of learning which stems largely from a cognitivist perspective. For example, Burnard and Chapman (1990) and Byran (1991) discuss how theories and concepts of student-centred learning in nurse education are underpinned by cognitivist theory and Bruner's theories in particular. Therefore in this literature review, as the concept of learner-centredness is the focal issue, a broadly cognitivist type perspective will form part of the theoretical framework.

Student-centred learning and teaching in nurse education

Bevis and Murray (1990), Burnard (1986b), Coombe et al (1981), French and Cross (1992), Gott (1982), Hurst (1985), and Sweeney (1986) describe traditional nurse education as being teacher-centred and pedagogical in orientation. In contrast, progressive nurse education is described as being student-centred and andragogical in orientation (Hurst 1985).

There is a wealth of literature in the field of nurse education which advocates a student-centred approach or progressive orientation in nurse education programmes. Much North American literature relating to nurse education over the last decade has had learner-centredness as a focal issue (Coombe et al 1981, Chally 1992, Bevis and Murray 1990, Di Rienzo 1983, Nielsen 1992, Pugh 1976, Tanner 1990). In the United Kingdom similar interests can be demonstrated (Beckett & Wall 1985, Bell 1984, Brookes et al 1983, Burnard 1985, Burnard 1989a, Carter 1979, Chiarella 1988, Crout 1980, Duffy 1985, Goodall 1985, Hurst 1985, Jarvis 1992a, Richardson 1988, Sweeney 1986, Webb 1979). For example, in the United Kingdom context Burnard and Chapman 1990 epitomise this advocacy of student-centred learning by saying:

> that the accent in nurse education should be towards the educational encounter being student-centred rather than teacher-centred and appropriately adult-centred. (p.65)

In the literature reviewed there was no literature found which explicitly questioned the educational value of adopting a learner-centred approach in nurse education.

There has, however, been limited research conducted into learner-centredness of nurse education programmes in the United Kingdom. For example, Alexander (1984) conducted a survey of pre-registration student nurses' (n=118) experiences of clinical teaching. It was concluded that much of the teaching was conducted by ward staff whose earlier experiences of nurse education had been of a passive nature, with an accent on didactic forms of teaching. However, although these conclusions were hypothesised by Alexander, their validation was not sought in the research conducted.

Gott (1982) in a comparative observational study of classroom teaching sessions (125 sessions were observed), used as a sample pre-registration nursing students in three schools of nursing. It was found there was little evidence of application of student-centred approaches and the main teaching format used was the traditional lecture method. However, Clarridge et al (1992) conducted a similar study to that of Gott's but used a post-registration student group as a sample and non-comparative quantitative methodologies (teaching sessions were observed over a two week period). They found that a high degree of learner-centred approaches were used.

The concept of adult learning and validity of use of chronological stages in learning will be examined in more depth at a later point in this literature review, however, it is appropriate at this point to identify the differences in pre-registration and post-registration nurse training with regard to these findings. Recruitment profiles show that there is still an outstanding need to recruit more mature entrants, those from ethnic minorities and males into nursing in Great Britain. The 'average' nursing recruit's profile continues to be that of a young, white and female (Casey and Buchan 1989, Hanson and Patchett 1986, Lathlean 1987). However, Miers (1992) states that the needs of mature pre-registration nursing students differ from those of younger pre-registration nursing students. In the very limited context of the studies of Gott (1982) and Clarridge et al (1992) it would seem that there is a small amount of evidence that pre- and post-registered courses do differ in their learner-centredness. Therefore there is also the implication that teaching young and older adults in nursing needs to viewed differently.

Sweeney (1990) conducted a comparative study of the learner-centredness of two registered general and two registered mental health nursing courses as perceived by third year student nurses. The research tool utilised was Boydell's Scale for Measuring the Learner-Centredness of a Course. Sweeney found first-level courses were generally highly teacher-centred in terms of planning, direction, sequence, pace and evaluation of learning. The climate of learning was moderately learner-centred, though teacher-student relationships were perceived as formal. A significantly higher level of perceived learner-centredness was found with regard to the of mental health courses studied.

A further point can therefore be drawn from the limited findings of Sweeney's (1990) coupled with those of Gott (1982) and Clarridge et al (1992). Not only may there be differences in pre- and post-registration courses' learner-centredness but there may also be differences in learner-centredness with regard to the type of pre-registration training which is being undertaken. These studies into learner-centredness, however, have a number of individual methodological weaknesses. For example, all have relatively small samples taken from limited locations in the United Kingdom. The validity of the findings is therefore low. However, a more fundamental weakness is that of the nature of the research questions. For example, learner-centredness as referred to earlier is a broad concept which may incorporate differing facets of meaning. To conduct meaningful research into a multi-faceted concept is a difficult endeavour, which is perhaps why there is only very limited research into the topic. Therefore in order to explore the pertinent literature further a more precise definition is needed.

A number of authors have linked the tenets inherent in the concept of andragogy with learner-centredness (Burnard 1985, Happs 1991, Ho 1991, Myles 1991, Raudonis 1987). Burnard, for example, relates that many writers use the concepts felt to be inherent in an andragogical approach as being synonymous with student-centredness. Therefore in the following section the concept of andragogy will be explored in order to provide a more exact definition and a subsequent framework for the first part of this literature review.

Concept of andragogy

Mazhindu (1990) recounts that the term andragogy was a word first used by the Yugoslav adult educator Dusan Savisevic and was later developed as a theory by Knowles (1970). Andragogy refers broadly to the art and science of helping adults learn and pedagogy to the art and science of helping children to learn. In Knowles' early work clear distinctions are made between the learning and teaching implications of the chronological andragogy and pedagogy models proposed.

Knowles I (1970) early distinction between pedagogy and andragogy, however, has generated much academic debate. For example, Jarvis (1986) states that initially

McKenzie (1977) sought to provide Knowles' pragmatic formulation with a more substantial philosophical base and argued that adults and children are existentially different. Elias (1979), however, argued that men and women are different but there has been no suggestion that teaching women is different than teaching men. As Jarvis points out, McKenzie assumed without empirical evidence that children are not as ready to learn as adults.

During this period of debate Knowles (1980) retracted his position and accepted there is not really a distinction by age in the concepts of andragogy and pedagogy but an inherent difference in approaches to teaching and learning. Knowles states pedagogical models refer to a content-based curriculum and andragogical models to a process-based curriculum. This point returns us then to the earlier debate on the nature of learning and learning theories. Knowles' later work referring to process-based educational theory in the context of adult education would seem to marry with theories of learning expounded by cognitivist theorists such as Bruner (1966) and concepts of progressive nurse education.

Whilst exploration of models of pedagogy fall outside the remit of this book and it is acknowledged that Knowles has not worked out systematically the implications of these distinctions, it would, however, seem, as Burnard and Morrison (1992) point out, that a more behaviourist orientation to teaching children is an implicit feature in Knowles' model of pedagogy and is also typified in traditional models of nurse education.

The development and debate regarding andragogical theory in wider educational circles is reflected in the nurse education context. For example, Beeman (1988), Burnard (1986b), French and Cross (1992), Matzhindu (1990), Pinkney-Atkinson (1983), Sweeney (1986) and Whittaker (1984) define andragogy as the art and science of helping adults learn, which can be contrasted to pedagogy or the art and science of teaching children. In giving these definitions there is acceptance of distinct differences between the teaching and learning of children and adults.

Burnard and Morrison (1992), Happs (1991), Ho (1991), Jarvis (1986), Myles (1991) and Raudonis (1987) are authors in nurse education who refer to the wider debate regarding chronological distinctions and their relevance to teaching and learning. Myles, for example, suggests that andragogy is an ideology rather than a theory of adult education and that it is a term given to an expanding body of knowledge of how adults learn. Myles goes on to state that, whilst assumptions that pedagogy differs from andragogy in terms of chronological development issues are suspect and may relate to differing learning philosophies, the tenets of andragogy can be regarded as principally self-evident.

Happs (1991), Ho (1991) and Raudonis (1987), however, take a differing viewpoint to Myles (1991). For example, Raudonis and Ho refer to differences in the learning and teaching of adults and children in terms of social roles and status. The teaching of adults, it is argued, needs to be based on differing principles because of these diversities. Happs also acknowledges that adult learning theory may be based in part on social perspectives of the role and status of adults in society but, using the work of Riegel (1973), conceptualizes adulthood as a further period of cognitive growth. Happs hypothesizes that further cognitive structural changes do occur in adulthood and are exemplified by development of the dialectical logic of mature thought. Dialectic thinking is demonstrated by discovering important questions and problems rather than by determining answers. Therefore adulthood from these view points is seen as differing from childhood both quantitatively and qualitatively.

Having examined some of the theories and debates surrounding the concept of andragogy, the following section of this chapter will examine definitions of andragogy and how these have been interpreted in the arena of nursing education.

Definitions of andragogy

A definition of andragogy as an ideology rather than theory is implicit in the work of Mezirow (1981). For example, Mezirow sees andragogy as a professional perspective of adult educators and offers a charter of andragogy for adult educators. The charter is based on a definition of andragogy as being:

> an organised and sustained effort to assist adults to learn in such a way that enhances their capability to function as self-directed learners. (p.21)

The beliefs of Knowles (1980) and the definition and charter proposed Mezirow (1981) regarding andragogy have been incorporated into assumptions nurse educators have regarding nursing education. For example, Burnard (1986b), Mazhindu (1990), Myles (1991), Nielsen (1992), Orr (1990) and Whittaker (1984) identified four basic tenets upon which andragogical nurse education should be based. These are as follows:

1. A change in self-concept from one of total dependence to increasing self-directedness.
2. Previous life experiences mean individuals become a rich resource for teaching, while providing a broadening base to which to relate new learning.
3. A readiness to learn, based upon need, in preparation for developing professional roles.
4. An orientation to learning, that of a problem-solving approach, which utilises the desire to apply learning to current situations.

Rachal and DeCoux (1992), in a review of literature pertaining to andragogy in a nursing context, conclude that andragogy can be seen to be a currently favoured ideology in nurse education. Rachal and DeCoux go on to state that few commentators and researchers have examined nursing education philosophy from an adult education perspective. In a North American study Hopkins (1981) and McKenzie (1987), however, have attempted to do this and they suggest that adult education philosophy and values are not deeply embedded in nursing educational philosophy. A similar point was raised earlier in this literature review in the context of the behaviourist/cognitive dichotomy.

A focal point of the first part of this literature review is therefore to utilise an adult educational and cognitivist-type perspective to evaluate the extent to which these philosophies are inherent in nurse educational research and literature. A further feature of the review will be assessment of the value of learning and teaching methods advocated by an andragogical perspective. The framework of the following sections of this chapter will therefore utilise the definition of andragogy given previously. Articulation of this definition is seen as being the use of self-directed, experiential and problem-solving learning and teaching methods in nurse education. These areas may also be identified as important in cognitive-type learning theories. For example, Bruner (1966) identifies similar areas of concern in terms of emphasising active restructuring of knowledge through experience with the environment. Also that learners should organise knowledge for themselves by, for example, using discovery methods rather than having material pre-packaged by the teacher.

The framework utilised for the review of the literature pertaining to student-centred learning and teaching and concepts of andragogy is given in the figure 2.1.

```
                    > Self-               > Development of
                    > Directed            > Self-Directed
                    > Learning            > Learning Skills
                    > and                 >       |
                    > Teaching            > Learning Styles
Student-            >    |                >       |
Centred             >    |                > Learning Preferences
Learning            >    |                >       |
and                 >                     > Contract Learning
Teaching            > Experiential        >       |
    |               > Learning and        > Reflective Learning
Andragogical        > Teaching            >       |
Concepts            >    |                > Negotiation and Use
                    >    |                > of Experiential
                    >    |                > Learning and Teaching
                    >    |                >       |
                    >    |                >       |
                    > Problem-solving     > Development of
                    > Learning and        > Critical Thinking
                    > Teaching            > Skills
                    >                     >
```

Figure 2.1 **Flow chart of the major topics reviewed in the literature pertaining to student-centred learning and teaching and concepts of andragogy**

Manifestations of student-centred learning and teaching and andragogical assumptions in nurse education

It has been identified that the assumptions inherent in the concept of andragogy will form the framework for this section of the literature review. The concept of andragogy is a focal issue as it is purported to be an approach which gives unification and articulation to learner-centredness in nursing education. As discussed previously, the tenets of Knowles' (1980) model of andragogy in nursing education relate to an increasing need of adults to be self-directed learners who utilise personal experience to modify their self-concept, and who use a problem-solving and inductive reasoning approach to learning. Therefore it is in this context that the following sections of the literature review will examine and evaluate teaching and learning methods used to assess and develop self-directed learning abilities in nursing students.

Self-directed learning in nurse education

Definitions of self-directed learning

Knowles (1975) defines self-directed learning as:

> a process in which individuals take the initiative, with or without help of others, in designing their learning needs, formulating learning goals, identifying human and material resources for learning, choosing and implementing appropriate learning strategies and evaluating learning outcomes. (p.8)

This definition enlarges on the central aim of education given by, for example, Bruner (1966), which is to make learners self-sufficient. The inter-relationships between cognitivism and andragogy also are further demonstrated by Shane (1983), who states that as one matures self-concept moves from total dependency to increasing self-directedness and adults will therefore resist learning under conditions that are incongruent with their self-concepts as autonomous individuals.

In a nursing context Wiley (1983) identifies two dimensions to self-directed learning. Self-directed learning is defined as activities in which learners takes the initiative and responsibility for learning processes and assumes control over most of the learning variables. However, a further dimension is added by Wiley, namely other-directed learning. Whilst participation in these activities is initially instigated by learners' objectives, resources and activities are controlled by others. Examples of these activities are given as attendance at conferences, courses and workshops. Whilst it is recognised that both these dimensions are of importance in nurse education the emphasis will be on the first dimension given by Wiley as the latter is seen as being of only peripheral importance to this literature review.

The relevance of self-directed learning in nursing

A number of authors in nursing education refer to the need for nurses to be self-directed learners (Clarke 1986, Coombe et al 1981, Crook 1985, Iwasiw 1987, Jarvis 1987, Jones 1980, O'Kell 1988, Prociuk 1990 St Claire and Brillhart 1990 Wiley 1983). For example, Jarvis and O'Kell state that it is increasingly necessary for nurses to view learning as a lifelong activity. This is seen as of importance when viewed in the context of, for example, the account given by Schoen (1979), who states that the volume of scientific knowledge has been estimated to be doubling itself every twenty years. Nursing therefore can expect rapid changes to professional practice in the future. Simpson (1979), however, recounts that many British nurses appear to believe that the skills and knowledge acquired during initial education programmes provide them with an adequate basis for life-long professional practice. However, the proposals of The Report of the Post Registration Education and Practice Project (UKCC 1991) may be seen to incorporate a professional requirement for continuing professional education to be viewed as life-long activity for all practitioners.

Nurses as self-directed learners

A number of North American studies have compared attitudes of nurses to self-directed learning with attitudes of other professional groups. For example, Linares (1989) compared attitudes of nursing students (n=170) and generic baccalaureate students (n=175). Measuring instruments used were the Adult Nowicki-Strickland Internal-External Scale, Guglielmino's Self-Directed Learning Readiness Scale and Rezler's Learning Preference Inventory. Findings of the study reveal no differences between the groups studied. However, significant differences in regard to age were demonstrated in that the older the student the higher the Self-Directed Learning Readiness score. Oddi (1988) conducted a similar study to that of Linares (1989). The sample for the study was graduate students in nursing (n=78), law (n=llO) and adult education (n=83). A multi measurement approach was again used. Significant differences were found with regard to nursing students obtaining higher scores on the Commitment to Learning scale. Livneh (1988) also examined human service professionals' (n=253) attitudes to self-directed learning and found that educability was the greatest predictive factor for forecasting the number of hours spent in self-directed learning activities. Educability in this study was defined as an interest in reading constituting appropriate self-directed learning skills.

Studies have also been conducted in North America analysing self-directed learning practices or how many hours nurses spend in self-directed study activities. Dixon (1991) investigated amounts of time Registered Nurses (n=99) spend on various kinds of self-directed learning projects. Using Guglielmino's Self-Directed Learning Readiness Scale it was found the sample had higher scores on learning-readiness than did adults in the general population. High scores were also correlated with above average amounts of time spent on self-directed professional learning. Emblen and Gray (1990) also compared how many hours baccalaureate-prepared nurses (n=40) and master's-prepared nurses (n=40) spent on self-directed learning. It was found that master's-prepared nurses spent more time per year on independent learning projects and slightly more time studying professional issues.

How nurses view themselves as self-directed learners has also been the focus of a number of studies, again in North America. For example, St Clair and Brillhart (1990) evaluated a self-directed learning programme which assessed self-directed learning readiness in a sample of 45 qualified nurses. Using Guilielmino's scale it was found that 62% of the sample rated themselves above the mean as self-directed learners.

There are, however, a number of problems in drawing generalised conclusions from findings of these studies. For example, Clarke (1986) and Emblen and Gray (1990) state that self-directed learning habits of nurses have not been widely addressed in research projects pertaining to nurse education. Also all the studies reviewed have been conducted in North America so applicability to other countries may be questionable. That relatively few studies have been conducted with small samples sizes implies that the validity of making generalisations from these findings is dubious.

A more fundamental critique may, however, also be made in that the majority of studies reviewed have taken as their research methodology perspective a broadly 'scientific' positivistic approach. Polit and Hungler (1991) describe problems inherent with this approach. For example, whilst biological and physical functioning is regular and consistent and less susceptible to external influences, human behaviour is influenced by a myriad of external variables. These variables include individual personalities, social environment, mental capacities, values, beliefs and lifestyles which collectively imply the essential uniqueness of individuals. Therefore in research terms difficulties arise when attempts are made to measure human behaviour. The validity of research tools for measuring attitudes and behaviour must be called into question. Also control of external variables may be seen as being fraught with difficulties.

With these reservations in mind it can, however, be seen that a number of the findings give limited validation to the tenets embedded in the concept of andragogy. For example Linares' (1989) findings demonstrate chronological differences in attitudes to self-directed learning. However, the findings of Livneh (1988) and Emblen and Gray (1990) give evidence that previous levels of educational achievement may be another important factor in determining attitudes to self-directed learning.

There is, however, conflicting evidence as to whether or not nurses are motivated to self-directed learning. For example, whilst Linares (1989) reported no differences, Dixon (1991) and Oddi (1988) do identify differences. Tough (1971) states that it common for a person to spend 700 hours a year in self-directed learning projects. In the studies reviewed estimates are given 370 hours (Dixon 1991) and 312 hours (Emblen and Grey 1990). Moreover Barnett (1981) and Stodulski and Stafford (1982) give evidence that nurses rarely read professional journals and Myco (1980) claims that nurses are unskilled in library use. It may therefore be concluded from this limited evidence that nurses do not spend as much time on self-directed learning projects as compared with the general population. The St Claire and Brillhart (1990) study, however, does give some evidence that nurses evaluate their self-directed study abilities as being high.

Self-directed learning readiness

There has been interest shown in estimating nursing students' readiness for self-directed learning. For example, O'Kell (1988) in a study in Britain used Guglielmino's Self-Directed Learning Readiness Scale (SDLRS) to test a group of 158 pre-registration nursing students. It was found that mean SDLRS scores fell with each successive year of training. It was therefore concluded 'that traditional nurse education trains out the quality of independence in students'.

Crook's (1985) study gives a further example of nurse educators' interest in self-directive learning readiness but in a North American context. Crook also used Guglielmino's scale and tested SDLRS scores and compared these with end of year assessment grades. The sample used was 63 pre-registration students in a baccalaureate programme at one Faculty of Nursing. There was found to be a weak but significant correlation between SDLRS scores and overall peer nomination in the first year. Peer nomination refers to students in the sample being asked to nominate the three 'most effective' self-directed learners in their tutorial group. However, it was concluded from the findings taken from previous year's scores that the SDLRS scale was not useful in predicting success of failure amongst the nursing students tested.

Crook (1985), however, identifies a number of methodological weaknesses in Guglielmino's scale. For example, peer nomination techniques had to be used as 'standard' and there are no 'golden standards' for the scale. It was also identified that no intra-rater or inter-rater reliability tests have been done on the SDLRS. Field (1989) also examines the structure, validity and reliability of Guglielmino's scale and concludes that there are major problems with wording used on the scale. Brockett 1985), moreover, comments that because of the terminology used the scale is not suitable for use with low-achieving adults. In addition Field states that there are serious flaws with developmental concepts which underpin the structure of the scale. Therefore the findings of Crook, of O'Kell (1988) and previously described studies which have utilised this scale may have possible weaknesses in term of validity and reliability of findings.

Iwasiw (1987) researching in a similar area, however, used qualitative methodology and recounts that assessing students' readiness for assuming responsibility for their learning activities should fall within the general remit of teachers when teaching. Iwasiw describes how question and answer sessions can help teachers assess an individual student's readiness to learn. An example is given of direct questioning about students' past learning experiences and how this may elicit unrecognised examples of self-directed learning. However, whether teachers do actually use these techniques was not empirically tested by Iwasiw and no further studies have been uncovered into this subject area.

Learning how to learn

Interest has also been focused on 'learning how to learn' study programmes as a teaching method to develop skills required to be self-directed when undertaking learning activities (Brookes et al 1983, Coombe et al 1981, Jarvis 1992b, Jones 1980, Schmidt and Fisher 1993, Wiley 1983).

Jones (1980) in the United Kingdom describes development of a module in a pre-registration nurse education course which was based on developing learning skills required for self-directed learning. The approach Jones describes has student selected goals of learning as a focal issue. However, no empirical evaluation of its learning effectiveness is given. Brookes et al (1983) also describe a similar approach taken with post-registration students on a nursing management course. However, again no empirical evaluation of its learning effectiveness is given. Similarly Schmidt and Fisher (1993) describe the development of self-study material aimed to enhance learning skills required for self-directed learning but do not give an evaluation of its effectiveness.

Wiley (1983) in the North American context has, however, conducted an empirical study into the effectiveness of a preparation programme for self-directed learning. The sample was baccalaureate nursing students and were divided into a control group of 50 and an experimental group of 54. Guglielmino's scale was utilised as the measurement tool of SDLR. Findings of the investigation suggest that teaching self-directed study skills did not significantly increase the students' ability to direct their own learning when compared with the control group. However, both control and experimental groups did gain on their SDLR scores.

There are, however, some methodological weaknesses inherent in Wiley's (1983) study. For example, Guglielmino's SDLRS scale was used to assess students readiness for self-directed study. A critique of this scale has been given at an earlier point in this chapter. Also the study used a relatively small sample of students from one location, which implies that the reliability and predictive validity of the findings is low. This critique of Wiley's study coupled with the lack of empirical evidence of the other studies reviewed therefore infers that effectiveness of learning how to learn programmes in nursing education cannot be demonstrated in the studies included in this literature review.

The learning effectiveness of self-directed study programmes

There have been a number of studies which have focused on establishing the educational effectiveness of self-directed study programmes. For example, in a North American context Hegge (1985) gives a model of continuing nursing education through self-directed learning. Prociuk (1990) conducted a study which evaluated self-directed learning approaches and their effectiveness in hospital orientation programmes. Findings show that Registered Nurses (n=150) in the study preferred to use self-directed learning over learning directed by educators. Flewellyn and Gosnell (1985) conducted a similar study which compared two approaches to hospital orientation programmes for practice efficacy and preferred learning methods of

Registered Nurses (n=110). It was found in the study that the group undertaking the competency-based programme (n=49), which consisted of self-selected learning material and teaching methods demonstrated more learning of subject areas covered than the group who undertook a traditional teacher-centred orientation programme (n=61). Finally Miller (1982) studied self-directed learning with regard to community need assessment. It was hypothesized that the more students test out their own ideas the better is the learning that takes place. However, the hypothesis was not empirically tested.

From a differing perspective Craig and Page (1982) describe the effectiveness of self-directed post-clinical conferences in terms of teacher performance (n=14). It was found that this approach generated an improvement not only in student participation but also in teachers demonstrating higher level questioning skills as measured on Bloom's taxonomy.

In the United Kingdom there have been few reported studies of the learning effectiveness of self-directed study programmes. D'A Slevin and Lavery (1991) in a similar context to Hegge (1985) describe how self-directed learning approaches can be incorporated into pre-registration programmes but like Hegge they give no empirical evidence of their effectiveness. However, Logue (1984) does describe the development of guided study units in an introductory course on anatomy and physiology. Evaluation of the study unit's effectiveness was conducted through student evaluations and examination pass rates. It was concluded by Logue that although there were some disadvantages to the introduction of this method of learning generally it was more effective than previous teacher-centred approaches. Brookes (1991) in a similar study to Logue describes the introduction of self-study anatomy and physiology and mental health law programmes in a pre-registration mental health nurse training curriculum. In a three year study of the implementation of these programmes post-test scores for the trial groups showed substantially better mean scores than for baseline groups.

Parfitt (1989) also describes an empirical study conducted in the United Kingdom the purpose of which was to see if creative teaching methods as against didactic teaching would prove effective when included in a School of Nursing teaching programme. The creative teaching methods Parfitt describes are those of self-directed studying. The sample was student nurses (n=80) in four introductory courses in two Schools of Nursing. Multiple-choice objectives tests, essay questions and assessment of practical skills were used to measure student learning outcomes. The findings show that the experimental group did no better in objective tests or in essays but did significantly better in problem identification and planning for nursing intervention.

It may therefore be concluded from these few studies reviewed into self-directed learning projects that their educational effectiveness may have some limited validation. However Logue (1984) reports some students did not like self-directed methods of study as they found them lonely and boring. A central point is therefore that account needs to be taken of individual differences in learning or how learning is best achieved for individuals. This focus will be considered in depth in the following chapter of this literature review in terms of individuality of patient care or how andragogical principles applied in a nurse education context relate to the delivery of patient care. However, the following section will focus on manifestations of individuality in nurse education or how self-directed learning strategies take account of differences in learning styles and learning preferences.

Learning styles

O'Kell (1988) identifies that there may be links with self-directed or learning prone personalities and students' learning style categories. Partridge (1983), however, describes the complexities of the subject area and identifies that in general education research has focused on two broad areas, those of cognitive style and student response styles. Much research in nurse education has, however, had as its focal point assessment cognitive learning styles and has concentrated on psychological testing of nurses' learning styles (DeCoux 1990, Dux 1989, Hodges 1988, Laschinger and Boss 1984, Laschinger 1986, Linares 1989, Merritt 1983, Norris 1986, O'Kell 1988, Partridge 1983, Schare et al 1991, Stevenson 1986). In particular interest has focussed on Kolb's (1976).

DeCoux (1990) reports that, although there are a large number of instruments available, Kolb's Learning Style Inventory (LSI) is the instrument used most frequently for measuring the learning styles of nurses. DeCoux identifies the learning styles in Kolb's (1976) model as follows:

1 Divergers, who excel in concrete experiences and reflective observational abilities. These learners are described as being people-orientated.
2 Accommodators, who excel in concrete experience and active experimentation skills. These learners are people-orientated and active learners.
3 Convergers, who excel in abstract conceptualization and active experimental skills. Whilst less people-orientated, they are good at applying theory to practical situations.
4 Assimilators, who excel in abstract conceptualization and reflective observational skills. They are less people-orientated and less practical than other learners.

Laschinger (1986) in a North American study examined learning characteristics of incoming student nurses (n=166). It was found that the majority of students had diverger-type learning styles (n=52) or accommodator-type learning styles (n=46). However, there were representatives of all types of learning styles in the sample (converger-type learning styles n=40 and assimilator n=28). In contrast O'Kell (1988) in the United Kingdom found in a similar study that 70% of a sample of student nurses (n=158) were either convergers or accommodators. Hodges (1988) also found from a sample of similar characteristics (n=62) that the majority were either convergers or accommodators. However, both O'Kell and Hodges found substantial representation in their samples of other types of learning styles.

The limited findings of these studies can be given as evidence that nurses cannot be conceived as a homogeneous group and that individual differences in learning styles may exist in any group of nurse learners. However, problems may be identified with these findings. For example, in a similar context to previously given criticisms of

Guglielmino's scale there are criticisms of Kolb's scale. O'Kell (1988), for example, reports that there were substantial problems with respondents' interpretation of the scale, and some respondents described the scale as confusing, vague and obscure. DeCoux (1990) also states that Kolb postulates that individuals with certain learning styles gravitate towards certain careers. Albeit that a relatively few studies have been reviewed, all the studies show that nursing students are represented in all four learning styles. Therefore one of Kolb's basic premises cannot be shown to be validated in the literature reviewed.

Learning preferences

Loesch and Foley (1988) identify differences between learning style or the manner in which a person perceives and processes information in a learning situation and learning preference, which is defined as the choice of one learning situation over another.

Merritt (1983) in a North American study used Kolb's LSI to assess its relationships to age and professional nursing experience of baccalaureate registered nurses (n=216) and nursing students (n=127). Findings for both groups of learners supported propositions that age and length of career employment account for differences in ways adults prefer to learn. For example, Registered Nurses in the sample were positively orientated to learning in formal settings but preferred to be actively involved in learning.

Baldwin et al (1991) and McAdam et al (1989), also in North America, investigated learning preferences in clinical skills training laboratories. McAdam et al, using a sample of baccalaureate student nurses (n=59) found use of a self–directed learning methodologies was supported by students studied. Baldwin et al compared two teaching strategies in a similar scenario (n=17). The strategies were a self–directed study approach and teacher–centred instruction. It was found that, whilst outcome measures for the two approaches were little different, mediated instruction was not appropriate as a complete substitute for teacher contact.

Studies in the United Kingdom have also concentrated on learning preferences of nurses. For example, Dux (1989) undertook a comparative survey of Registered Nurses and Enrolled Nurses (n=119) attending courses at one College of Nursing in the United Kingdom and examined learning preferences of the sample. Both groups of students expressed preferences for active learning teaching methods. Teacher–centred methods such as, for example, lectures rated low on lists of preferred learning activities.

Vaughan (1990) conducted a similar study which investigated attitudes of general and mental health pre–registration student nurses (n=203) from nine Schools of Nursing in the United Kingdom. Vaughan found that there were few differences in the groups studied and students were more predisposed towards student–centred teaching and learning methodologies. Burnard and Morrison (1992) conducted similar research in a survey of nurse teachers and pre–registration students from 14 differing locations in the United Kingdom. The findings of this study, however, contrast with those of Dux and Vaughan in that the lecturers were more supportive of student–centred teaching and learning approaches than were students.

Ostrow (1986) and Fell (1989) investigated the use of an instruction method, Keller's Personalized System of Instruction, which is directed towards tailoring teaching approaches to be deployed to the individual needs of students. Both studies employed a comparative experimental approach. Ostrow's sample was undergraduate student nurses (n=75) and Fell's was beginner student nurses (n=43). Both researchers had control groups who undertook a lecture–type programme and experimental groups where the Keller method was utilised. Both studies used student evaluations and assessment of learning as measures of learning effectiveness. The findings of the studies show significant differences between the control group and experimental group. Use of the Keller Plan was demonstrated to be a more effective and preferred instructional method.

Learning style and learning preference

A number of authors have, however, concentrated upon links between learning style and learning preference. For example, Stevenson (1986) describes implementation of a new pre–registration nursing curriculum in the United Kingdom and how individual learning preferences and learning styles of students were a central focus. It was hypothesised that the minority of students would have learning preferences for teacher–centred activities and these would relate to differences in learning style. However, no systematic collection of empirical evidence of preferred learning activities or their relationship to learning styles is reported. McMillan and Dwyer (1990) in a similar context also suggest a facilitative approach to teaching and advocate matching teaching and learning styles.

In an empirical study in North America Brudenell and Carpenter (1990) utilised Kolb's Learning Style Inventory and investigated the relationship between learning styles of baccalaureate nursing students and attitudes towards a commuter-assisted instruction programme (CAI). Using Kolb's Learning Style Inventory, which again showed substantial representation in all learning style categories, attitudes to CAI were investigated. It was found that there were significantly negative attitudes towards the programme and this was irrespective of individual learning styles.

It may therefore be concluded from the limited findings of these studies that nursing students may on balance have a preference for student–centred teaching methodologies and therefore the implementation of certain andragogical tenets is validated. Also nurses are not a homogeneous group in terms of learning style categories.

There are, however, as reported in previous sections of this chapter, individual weaknesses in the studies reviewed in terms of their reliability and validity. Partridge (1983) also outlines why caution may need to be exercised when adopting student–centred approaches. Partridge states that whilst it may be sensible to match a student's preferred learning style with a congruent instructional mode, this assumes that students habitually utilise only one learning style. As with previous studies reviewed measurement of attributes and attitudes, in this instance learning styles and learning preferences, is only valid at a given point in time. In a similar vein to the previous critique of positivism Burnard (1992a) claims that people are dynamic in nature and ever–changing. Also it is suggested that, when attempting to match a student learning style or preferred learning methods with teaching methods, the purpose of educational endeavours must be identified. The question is therefore posed: is the purpose of education to learn subject matter or is the purpose developmental and to broaden students' learning potential?

In the following section of this literature review contract learning will be examined as an approach which may be seen to mitigate criticisms regarding learning styles and learning preferences.

Contract learning

Contract learning is identified by a number of authors as being a further dimension in the application of andragogical principles to nursing education (Clark 1990, Gibbon 1989, Keyzer 1986, Mazhindu 1990, Richardson 1987, Whittaker 1984, Wuest 1991). Richardson, for example, reports that learning contracts individualise teaching and learning processes and promote self–directedness and therefore assist students to develop habits related to life–long learning.

Learning contracts are defined by Gibbon (1989) as a:

> written agreement or commitment reached between a student and teacher regarding a particular amount of student work or learning and amounts of institutional reward or credit to be gained, this within a given time span. (p. 264)

Keyzer (1986) also emphasises that use of contract learning entails students being actively involved in learning and teaching processes. It is hypothesized that use of learning contracts results in students being intrinsically motivated to learning activities. This therefore develops a major feature of andragogical philosophy and, by giving primacy of importance of motivational factors, also matches with Bruner's perspective of the learning process.

A number of studies have investigated the use of contract learning. For example, Clark (1990) conducted a study in North America and compared traditionally-taught and learning-contract taught baccalaureate nursing students (n=86). Students' clinical performance scores and post self–directed learning readiness scores (using Guglielmino's SDLR scale) were compared. A significant relationship was found between mean scores in clinical performance and self–directed learning. These were found to be higher in the traditionally–taught groups. Wuest (1991), however, describes the introduction of contract learning as a vehicle for increased student involvement in audio teleconferencing. Contrary to Clark's report it was found that use of contract learning did increase students' self–directedness. Richardson (1988) also evaluated use of self–directed independent study contracts with pre–registration student nurses. It was found in an analysis of teacher activities prior to introduction of contract learning that learning activities were highly teacher–centred. Following the introduction of contract learning, teaching was more learner–centred.

A number of authors have examined the use of contract learning in the United Kingdom. For example, Gibbon (1989) describes introducing contract learning in an undergraduate pre–registration course. Student and teacher evaluations of the project were described as being favourable. Akinsanya (1987), Keyzer (1986) and Whittaker (1984) have conducted similar studies and their findings were analogous to those of Gibbon. Some disadvantages to contract learning are, however, identified by these authors. For example, Keyzer (1986) reports that implementation of contract learning relies upon a heavy time commitment from teachers. Gibbon (1989) also identifies that students' self–motivation is a crucial factor and hypothesizes that contract learning works better in small groups or in undergraduate courses. This again is because of the time–consuming element of contract learning. Also undergraduate student nurses are seen by Keyzer to be more intrinsically motivated to learning and to value independence more. A group of students (n=16) undertaking a post–registration Diploma in Nursing, however, have given an account of their own experiences of contract learning (Waltho 1986). The students concluded that contract learning 'challenged us and enhanced our will to learn'. The beliefs of Keyzer and the appropriateness of contract learning for undergraduate students would therefore appear to be contradicted by the report of Waltho.

The limited findings of these studies would seem on balance to vindicate use of contract learning in nurse education. Whilst disadvantages can be identified, it would appear that advantages outweigh these shortcomings. Contract learning can be seen to be highly student–centred and to permit identification of learning needs on an individual basis. However, as with previous studies reviewed the research methodologies utilised can be criticised. For example, with the exception of Clark's (1990) study all used a qualitative approach to data collection.

In a similar vein to the previously given critique of experimental methodologies, qualitative methodologies also have inherent weaknesses. Polit and Hungler (1991) state that qualitative methodologies have the advantages of being able to capture a direct record of behaviour and events and therefore give depth and variety of information. However with, for example, observational research methods disadvantages relate to perceptual errors and inadequacies. Observational bias may result in objectivity of data collection and analysis being sacrificed. Also the well recognised Hawthorne effect may affect individuals' behaviour and events. Similar criticisms may also be made to use of other qualitative research methods. For example, Polit and Hungler (1991) recount that collection of interview data depends quite heavily on the interpersonal skills of the interviewer. Major drawbacks are the potential for interviewer questions to bias responses.

It may, however, be summarised from the studies reviewed in this section of the literature review that there are numerous examples of advocacy of developing the self–directed learning skills of nurses. Also concepts, dimensions and application self–directed learning are complex and multi–faceted. Of the various dimensions explored, it may be concluded that certain tenets of andragogy are inherent in nurse education writers' and researchers' perspectives and these are integrally linked with a cognitivistic educational philosophy. There is, however, limited evidence of the educational effectiveness of application of such approaches.

In the following section of the literature review experiential learning and teaching will be examined and evaluated. This is in the context of andragogical principles of active learning, which utilises personal experiences to modify self–concepts and their contribution to the development of meaningful learning.

Experiential learning and teaching

Child (1986) states that cognitivistic perspectives of learning stress the importance of learning by insight or the fact that learners must have insight into the area of learning through personal experience. Understanding occurs through meaningful learning experiences. Boydell (1976), for example, draws a distinction between rote and meaningful learning. The outcome of rote learning using behaviourist principles of teaching and learning is the ability to recall or do things quickly and without thinking. As discussed in the introduction to this chapter, application of behaviourist theory and rote learning are seen by some as appropriate in certain areas of nurse education. Most notable of these areas is psychomotor skills training where the ability to perform tasks automatically is of importance. Meaningful learning, on the other hand, leads to understanding and the ability to make sense of things.

In a similar way to cognivist theory, concepts of andragogy have as a central feature previous life experiences which are seen as a rich resource for teaching and a base to which to relate new teaching. Both perspectives therefore have active learning as essential elements.

Definitions of experiential learning and teaching

Boydell (1976) offers a description of three types of experiential learning as follows:

Type 1: Gestalt–insight theories. In this theory learning occurs when a student who is faced with a problem restructures their perceptions in order to make sense of them. Suitable methods to facilitate this type of learning are questioning, discussions, case studies, role play, business games and structured experiments.

Type 2: Autotomous learning theory. Learning in this theory also occurs due to ways individuals restructure perceptions due to experience. Methodologies advocated are solving real or simulated problems and presented in a similar context to Type 1. It differs, however, from insight learning in that learners set their own goals, select and generate their own resources, and consider learning in terms of personal goals and feelings.

Type 3: Learning from everyday experiences. Everyday experience in this approach is equated to knowledge. Learning from everyday occupational experiences is therefore of importance.

In nurse education Burnard (1992a, 1992b and 1992c) examined student nurses' and nurse tutors' perceptions of experiential learning. In a survey (n=397) and interviews with student nurses (n=12), and nurse tutors (n=12) definitions of experiential learning were explored. Experiential learning and experiential learning methods were found to be used as synonyms. Boydell's Type 1 Gestalt–type experiential learning methods were clearly identified by both students and tutors. The tutors also described Boydell's Type 2 autonomous–type experiential learning. However, the students whilst recognising this dimension, felt it did not in actuality take place. Experiential learning was also identified as personal learning by both study groups, similar to Boydell's Type 3. The students studied, however, saw this type of experiential learning in terms of learning in clinical settings whereas the tutors identified it as occurring a classroom context.

In the following sections of this chapter these differing perceptions of experiential learning will be examined in the context of their manifestations in nurse education.

Experiential learning and teaching methods in nursing education

Many authors in nurse education advocate active classroom learning (Allcock 1992, Burnard 1988, Clark and Sleep 1990, Coombe et al 1981, Cotanch 1981, Dowie and Park 1988, Fowler et al 1987, Hamm and Brodt 1982, Hurst 1993, Leach 1988, Lopez 1983, Mander 1992, McCaugherty 1991a, Merchant 1989, Newsome 1983, Norris 1986, Parfitt 1989, Raichura 1987, Riseborough 1993, Schare et al 1991). Merchant (1989), for example, argues that the use of experiential methods are appropriate for teaching and learning in nurse education as learners need to be able to relate theory to practice in what is largely a practice discipline. In addition large amounts time are spent in clinical situations where it is assumed that many practical skills will be learnt.

There are a number of writers who give examples of adoption of experiential methods in learning and teaching of nurses. Allcock (1992) describes an experiential workshop used to teach patient assessment skills, Clark and Sleep (1990) demonstrate how research appreciation skills can be taught using group exercises for data collection, Burnard (1988) examines use of 'brainstorming' as a practical learning activity, Hamm and Brodt (1982) describe simulation and gaming as a way of teaching assertiveness skills, Hurst (1993) and Riseborough (1993) explore use of drama to teach family dynamics and health education, Leach (1988) describes an experiential approach to student nurse selection and Lopez (1983) and Raichura (1987) explore use of role play in teaching nurse–patient communication.

Evaluation of the use of these methods is not given by either Burnard (1988), Hurst (1993) or Raichura (1987). However, evaluations are given by Allcock (1992) and Lopez (1983), who report that the participating students thought it a valuable and worthwhile experience. Hamm and Brodt (1982) also report that preliminary findings indicate the teaching methods' effectiveness although there is no indication of how this was assessed. Similarly Leach (1988) recounts that wastage rates dropped but states that this cannot be claimed to be directly attributable to introducing experiential methods of selection.

Empirical research into the effectiveness of experiential learning methods has been conducted by Norris (1986) in a North American study. The study compared performance outcomes for groups of students (n=147) randomly assigned to role play or lecture instruction for learning basic communication skills. Overall test performance and ability to transfer content to practice did not differ between the two groups. However, it was found that the more mature the student the greater was the ability to transfer and apply communication concepts and skills. Smith (1982) also found that generally simulation gaming was less effective than conventional teaching methods in changing nurses' attitudes to perceptions of older people, but results differed according to the ages of the sample. Newsome (1983), however, found in a study of active learning versus lecture method that in a sample of 50 nursing students active learning was a more effective method in teaching students how to apply the nursing process. The measurement instrument used was Utilisation of the Nursing Process in Writing Care Plans.

It may be concluded from these few studies reviewed that experiential classroom learning methods are widely advocated in nurse education but that only limited research been conducted which validates their educational effectiveness. It is, however, seen as being a particular useful way by the majority of writers to bridge the so called theory:practice gap in nurse education. There is, however, little indication in any of the reports of negotiation or of the use of learning contracts when these methods were introduced.

Burnard (1989b) reports that there are numerous writings about experiential methods in nurse education but little reference to student choice regarding their use. He goes on to state that many adult educators argue that the individual's dignity and concept of self should be preserved but this is not always apparent when adopting the use experiential learning techniques. Also, as reported earlier, Shane (1983) states that adults will resist learning that is not congruent with their self–concept as autonomous individuals. Crout (1980), writing from a student nurse's viewpoint, says that often nurses in training are treated as unthinking children and in acceptance of the situation withdraw into apathy and non–response.

Negotiated experiential learning and teaching in nurse education

As discussed previously, there are few studies which focus on experiential learning based on negotiations and student choice. The earlier described studies of Dux (1989) and Vaughan (1990) can be given as evidence that student nurses prefer active learning methods as opposed to didactic teaching. Also Fowler et al (1987) describe from a student nurse's perspective an experiential learning episode when they decided to become elderly mentally ill patients for a day. Collectively the experience was seen as very traumatic but a worthwhile and interesting way to learn.

Facilitation of voluntary participation in experiential learning is explored by Dowie and Park (1988), who describe the use of a question–asking approach based on the work of Andrews' (1980). Questions regarding subject content of a lecture formed the focus of subsequent group work and discussion of real life issues. They describe how this method can facilitate voluntary contribution to an experiential element of a teaching session. Evaluations of the method is, however, not given.

In summary, no empirical evidence or evaluation has been found which addresses the question of whether or not student nurses voluntarily participate in experiential learning activities. This may be coupled with previous conclusions that there is also conflicting evidence regarding preferred learning activities.

Experiential learning and teaching and practical knowledge

The third area of experiential learning described by Boydell (1976) addresses everyday experiences as learning episodes. Nursing literature has long had as a focus case–study reports. For example, Mander (1992) describes how personal accounts of nurses' experiences in clinical settings appear frequently in the nursing press.

The work of Wood and Rubin (1992) can also be used as an example of this narrative or paradigm approach. They describe a case–study of an individual student nurse and subsequent decision–making processes regarding her future. Fieldhouse (1992) gives a further example of a nursing narrative in a clinical setting in describing the dilemma of caring for an elderly patient. Interestingly the dilemma centred on a care or not to care situation and the acknowledgement of the patient's individual right to choose or refuse to enter into a caring relationship. Whilst one example comes from a purely educational setting and the other a practice setting, similar concepts of autonomy and independence are addressed.

A number of studies have explored the contribution of personal experiences to learning nursing. For example, Mander (1992) in a study in the United Kingdom of midwifery care of mothers relinquishing babies for adoption found that the midwives attached considerable importance to learning from their past midwifery experiences. Occupational experience was seen to be of overwhelming significance.

McCaugherty (1991a), also in the United Kingdom, evaluated a teaching method based on discussions which centred on patients whom students had nursed. An experimental group (n=24) and control group (n=24) of student nurses were used as a sample. During clinical allocations the students were questioned regarding aspects of patient care they were nursing using a 'spot check' method. Twice as many students in the experimental group were found to be in a 'good' clinical skills category and twice many students in the control group were found to fall in the 'poor' clinical skills category.

In a similar North American study Di Rienzo (1983) employed the use of pre–clinical conferences in a baccalaureate nursing programme. It was found that content was related to practice more effectively and there were improvements in patient problem identification. Coombe et al (1981) also used a similar approach when teaching family dynamics to novice community health nurses. Students were, however, asked to apply a family assessment model to reflections on their own family backgrounds and life experiences rather than clinical scenarios. Written student evaluations were reported to be positive, although no evaluation is given of the efficacy of learning.

As discussed earlier in this review, experiential learning can be seen to encompass the dimension of learning in clinical practice. For example, Schumann (1990) in a North American survey of registered nurses (n=381) identifies that the nature and quality of clinical experience received the most frequent mention with regard to negative attitudes towards basic nurse training. Similarly Alexander (1984), in a study in the United Kingdom of student nurses' (n=119) preferences for methods of learning and teaching, found that ward tutorials and clinical teaching emerged as the clear favourites. Equally clear was the students' dislike of classroom teaching, whether or not this was experiential or didactic, self–directed or guided.

Criticisms of the research methods of these studies can be given in a similar way to those of previous studies. For example, all have relatively small samples taken from limited geographical locations. Reliability and validity of the findings may therefore be weak. Within these constraints, however, it can be concluded that learning from personal experiences has an overwhelming value in nurse education and this is particularly so of clinical experiences.

A number of authors, however, conclude that it is not the experience alone which results in meaningful learning but personal reflection on the experience or, in the context of nursing, reflection on professional experiences (Benner 1984, Burnard 1987, Jarvis 1992c, Schon 1983). Reflecting on personal experiences of nursing practice will therefore form the focus of the following section of this chapter.

Reflection on experiences of nursing

Learning through experience has been of central concern in the previous section of this literature review. Burnard (1987) drawing upon the work of Freire (1972) and Kolb (1984), however, describes the importance of learning not only through experience but from experience. Burnard reports that in learning from experience students are encouraged to reflect on past experiences as a means of discovering solutions to present problems from past situations. This reflective quality is also described by Freire, who believes that action without reflection does not lead to informed intentional behaviour whereas action followed by reflection can ensure that anything learned from the action can be carried forward to the next situation.

Jarvis (1992c) claims that, whilst no profession can be said to have reflective practice, it is possible to practise reflectively and that procedures should be laid down that encourage reflective or thoughtful practice. In this vein a number of writers describe the value of recording in a journal reflections on professional experiences.

Vaughan (1992), for example, describes the very personal experiences of a senior nurse's struggle to come to understand the nature of nursing knowledge through personal experiences of updating her clinical nursing skills. Cameron and Mitchell (1993) and Gallego and Walter (1991) outline the use of reflective journals in nursing education and describe how they facilitate students in taking an active role in the teaching and learning process. Jinks (1991) describes how nurse teachers can maximise the benefits of practical placements for students through encouraging reflection in and on practice in clinical teaching sessions. Finally Fabricius (1991) describes a project in which student nurses were offered the opportunity to belong to a small discussion group which met weekly during ward placements.

Of these studies reviewed, however, only Cameron and Mitchell (1993) and Fabricius (1991) offer evaluation of the use of reflective groups and journals. Fabricius found that use of reflective groups in student nurse education was expensive in teacher and student time. Whilst on average only a third of students wanted to participate in the groups, the depth of discussion gave the impression that their nursing practice would be affected. However, non–participating students tended to disparage the groups, conveying impressions that participants were non–copers and weak. Cameron and Mitchell (1993) also identify the possible misuse of reflective journals. For example, if journals are part of formal or informal assessment strategies this needs to be clearly identified. However, if journals are part of encouraging recordings of personal thoughts and reflections, confidentially must be maintained. In this situation the rights of students as free–thinking and autonomous individuals must be respected by the teachers involved.

In conclusion, it may be seen that experiential learning and application of experiential learning methods is, as with previous sections of this literature review, a complex and multi–faceted area of nursing education. However, notions of autonomy and independence on the part of student nurses appear to be of key significance in the literature reviewed. The effectiveness of teaching methods also is an important dimension, especially in relation to bridging the so called theory:practice gap in nursing education. The relationship between content and how that content is delivered, and relationships to clinical practice are therefore crucial issues.

The following section of this chapter will examine the final dimension of andragogy, namely that of an orientation to learning utilising a problem–solving approach.

Problem–solving teaching and learning in nurse education

In addressing the development of problem–solving abilities parallels between the tenets of andragogy and the skills necessary for providing effective nursing care can clearly be demonstrated. For example, Jones and Brown (1991) report that since the 1960's the nursing process has been the preferred method of providing professional nursing care. Hagell (1989) examined the underpinning assumptions of the nursing process and identified nursing's unique frame of reference for dealing with human problems. Nurses are said to have become increasingly aware that human interactions involve constant consideration of alternative possibilities. Moreover Jones and Brown consider that nursing decisions are explicated as the result of negotiation between alternative points of view, contradictory lines of reasoning and situational contingencies. Problem–solving or critical thinking skills are thus a focal ability in nursing decision–making in regards of patient care.

Definitions of critical thinking

Some theorists and researchers have characterized critical thinking as a unique cognitive process (Dewey 1933, Ennis 1985). Others have more narrowly defined critical thinking as a problem–solving technique which uses logical proposition (Siegel 1980, Ennis 1962). Dewey (1933), Ennis (1985) and Mezirow (1981), however, believe that critical thinking is grounded in reflective thought. For example, Mezirow (1981) extends the meaning of critical thinking from one that requires a correct assessment of statements to one that consists of a comprehensive process of reasonably and reflectively arrived at explanations.

Assessment of critical thinking skills in nursing students

A number of authors contend that nursing students are actively discouraged from questioning 'the facts' and are not taught to argue logically (Clinton 1985, Crout 1980, Sweeney 1986). Sweeney, for example, states that failure to develop independent, critical thinking abilities in nursing students leads to the perpetuation of professional decision–making on an 'ad hoc' or 'trial-and-error' basis. Decision–making is therefore based on rituals and routines and not on empirical research findings.

Gross et al (1987), however, in North America studied the impact of nursing education on students' critical thinking abilities. A sample of 108 associate and baccalaureate student nurses' critical thinking abilities were measured using the Watson–Glaser Critical Thinking Appraisal (WGCTA) instrument at entry to and exit from their programmes. It was found that all groups of students showed comparable improvement in critical thinking abilities.

Pardue (1987) also in a North American study investigated decision–making skills and critical thinking ability amongst associate degree, diploma, baccalaureate and master's prepared nurses (n=360). Instruments used were the WGCTA instrument and a researcher developed Decision–Making questionnaire. The findings show significant differences in critical thinking abilities in the sample. Baccalaureate- and master's-prepared nurses were found to have the highest mean scores of critical thinking abilities. These findings are congruent with the conclusions of Sparks (1982), who also found that baccalaureate and associate degree programmes prepare graduates to function differently in the area of problem–solving as demonstrated by the use of the nursing process.

Poole (1982), however, conducted a similar study to those of Pardue (1987) and Sparks (1982) and came to differing conclusions. Using as a sample 429 student from 13 nursing schools and also WGCTA scores, it was hypothesized that scores for both associate and baccalaureate degree students would rise following their course of studies. There was, however, no change over time in either group of students with regard to the low cognition dimension. Conclusions were drawn from the findings that traditional nurse educational methods and the teaching of the nursing process fostered logical (low cognition) rather than creative (high cognition) thinking.

Finally Kintgen–Andrews (1991) in a North American literature review examined the impact of nurse education on critical thinking abilities and the relationship between critical thinking and clinical judgement. On balance no strong support could be found for the statement that nurse education has a positive impact on the development of critical thinking skills. The studies reviewed that tested both critical thinking and clinical judgement provided practically no evidence of congruence between the two.

Applicability to other countries of these finding in respect of nurse education in the United Kingdom is clearly questionable. Very differing systems of nurse training mean generalisations from these research findings cannot be made. Also Bauwens and Gerhard (1987) in a North American study question the validity of the WGCTA instrument as a measure of the specific cognitive processes which underpin the use of the nursing process. For example, whilst their findings show WGCTA scores did correlate with examination success they did not, however, correlate with clinical practice grades.

Fewer research projects in this subject area have been conducted in the United Kingdom. Chang and Gaskill (1991) used Heppner et al's Problem–Solving Inventory to assess the attitudes of 67 pre- and post-registration nursing students towards problem–solving behaviour. It was found that there was no overall improvement in problem–solving behaviour over time although confidence in problem–solving had improved significantly.

Development of critical thinking skills in nursing students

The development of critical thinking skills and their relevance to the practice of nursing in the use of the nursing process has been the focus of an abundance of literature and research in nursing education. For example, Burnard (1988), Burnard (1989a), Peate (1992), Smith and Russell (1991) and Woolley (1990) describe strategies which are aimed at developing critical abilities in nursing students. Peate advocates the introduction debating forums, Burnard offers more general guidelines to nurse educators and the use of 'brainstorming' techniques and Smith and Russell advocate the use of critical learning experiences. Finally Woolley identifies the crucial interconnections between nursing's theoretical knowledge base and problem–solving. It is argued by Woolley that each of these distinct yet related domains must be addressed by the clinician when applying the reasoning process.

Empirical studies regarding evaluating critical thinking learning and teaching methods have also been conducted. For example, in North America Givens (1990) studied whether nurse educators could facilitate the cognitive development of baccalaureate nursing students by using writing strategies that challenged their thinking. Comparisons between an experimental group (n=29) and a control group (n=16) reveal, however, there were no significant differences between the two groups with regard to their cognitive and problem–solving abilities.

Lowdermilk and Fishel (1991), also in North America, examined the effectiveness of computer assisted instruction (CAI) as a measure of baccalaureate student nurses' decision–making skills (n=64). It was found that students who had higher scores on decision–making with regard to the CAI programme achieved higher clinical scores. However whether CAI helped students to achieve the higher clinical scores could not be demonstrated. Holzemer (1986) conducted a similar study the purpose of which was to explore the problem–solving skills of nurse practitioners (n=79). It was found that the sequence of subjects' movement through the clinical simulations was in close agreement with the optimal route given by the instrument author. However, when the subjects varied this route their performance was negatively affected. The subjects generally had a common sequential approach to the problem–solving task. Farrand et al (1982), however, found in a parallel study that there were significant differences between Registered Nurses and nurse practitioners' abilities. More experience of nursing was hypothesized to account for these differences.

Philosophies of the nursing process and applicability to critical thinking theories

In the introduction to this section of this literature review a description of the nursing process was given that is congruent with the broader definition of critical thinking as, for example, offered by Dewey (1933). However, an alternative perspective on the nursing process is offered by Jones and Brown (1991) which sees it as based on a rational–linear or scientific approach. Happs (1991) sees this perspective as being in accord with a reductionist mechanistic view of humans. Crudely the nursing process is a step by step approach to identification of nursing problems, initiation of problem–solving strategies and evaluation of these strategies. Whilst care is said to be individualised or tailored to meet the unique needs of individuals this is constrained by a mechanistic view of people. This logical rational perceptive is in keeping with the definitions of critical thinking as offered by Ennis (1962) and Siegel (1980).

Incorporation of the rational–logical perspective of the nursing process in nurse education, however, has the potential to create tension and conflict amongst competing philosophical viewpoints. For example the advocacy of this scientific logical method of care supports students reaching 'correct' solutions. However, critical thinking theory particularly and andragogical theory generally recognise the centrality of independent thought and action to substantive learning. There is also an orientation to cognition predicated upon reflective thought and a tolerance for ambiguity. In this perspective there is no one 'correct' solution because by using critical thinking processes legitimate but differing interpretations are possible. This view very much marries with the view of the uniqueness of individuals and their health and nursing needs. It can, however, be concluded that most of the published literature on critical thinking in nurse education takes a narrow mechanistic perspective on the nursing process.

Exploration of beliefs regarding the rational–linear or scientific nature of the nursing process by nurse teachers (n=40) is demonstrated in an empirical study by Sheahan (1991). Using a grounded theory approach in four schools of nursing in the United Kingdom Sheahan found that problem–solving was seen by the sample as characteristic of the nursing process approach. However, strong contrasts emerged in relation to the scientific standing of the nursing process and varying degrees of discord in relation to the individualised and systematic characteristics of this approach.

Similar criticisms may be made of Sheahan's (1991) study to those given to previously reviewed studies. However, Sheahan acknowledges that as far as he knows this is the first study to investigate formally the conceptual nature of the nursing process approach. Therefore, although tentative findings are given interesting possibilities emerge for future research in this area.

The theory:practice divide in nurse education

Much of this chapter has implicitly or explicitly addressed how teaching and learning methods in classroom environments can be seen to interrelate with the skills necessary for effective nursing practice. Effective nursing practice has been defined as that framed by use of the nursing process with an emphasis on providing individualised care or patient–centred care. The theory:practice gap in nursing has been an underlying issue. It is, however, also recognised that whilst the effectiveness of student–centred teaching and learning methods and their relationship to the skills and abilities necessary to provide professional nursing care are important, these form only part of a broader area of inquiry.

A number of authors, for example, have examined the relevance of curriculum structure to the theory:practice divide (Burrell 1988, Hawkett 1989, McCaugherty 1991b, Smith 1987, Webb 1989, Wong 1979), whilst others have explored the relationship of curriculum content and sequencing (Burrell 1988, Di Rienzo 1983, Frish 1988, Jacka and Lewin 1986, Mallick 1977, Pardue 1979, Smith 1992). The relevance of assessments has also been examined (Ashworth and Morrison 1991, Boreham 1977, Cameron and Mitchell 1993, Taylor 1991). Exploration of the effects of the hidden curriculum and occupational socialisation has also been the focus of attention (Baxter 1992, Bell 1984, Cook 1991, Crout 1980, Melia 1984). Liaison and involving clinical staff in curriculum development and delivery have also been topics of inquiry (Houston and Weatherston 1986, Stevenson 1985, Weatherston 1981). Finally, the changing the role of nurse teachers has also been addressed as providing solutions to the theory:practice divide (Alexander 1982, Chandler 1991, Clifford 1993, Crotty 1993a, Holloway and Penson 1987, Jarvis 1992a, Jinks 1991, Miller 1985, Vaughan 1989).

The majority of these studies, however, focus on the negative aspects of the theory:practice divide in nurse education and give possible solutions to narrowing that divide. In contrast, Lindsay (1990) explores the incompatibility between nursing theory and clinical nursing practice and suggests that nursing needs such a divide in order for theory to develop. For example, Lindsay advocates that theory should drive practice and in order for this to happen there will inevitably be a theory:practice gap. However, important for Lindsay is that all theory development should stem from practice–based research.

In conclusion, it is recognised that examination of these broader areas of inquiry into the theory:practice divide in nurse education in a discrete fashion fall outside the remit of this book. However, it is acknowledged that in general terms they impinge and have relevance to this literature review given in this chapter.

3 Patient–centred nursing care and student–centred learning and teaching

This chapter addresses the second stage of the literature review conducted and has patient–centred nursing care as a focus. The following flow chart gives the framework used for this section of the literature review. Identified are the concepts deemed as being of importance in regard to patient–centred nursing care and their inter–relationships with student–centred learning and teaching.

Patient–	>	Humanism	>			
Centred	>	¦	>			
Nursing	>	¦	>			Individualised
Care	>	¦	>	Personhood	>	Patient care
¦	>	¦	>	¦	>	¦
¦	>	¦	>	¦	>	¦
¦	>	¦	>	¦	>	Care and
¦	>	¦	>	¦	>	Care–Giving
¦	>	¦	>	¦	>	¦
Student–	>	¦	>	Development	>	¦
Centred	>	¦	>	of Self–	>	Power and
Learning	>	¦	>	Concept	>	Control
and	>	Effective	>		>	
Teaching	>	Teaching	>		>	
	>	Behaviour	>		>	

Figure 3.1 Flow chart of the major topics reviewed in the literature pertaining to patient-centred nursing care and student-centred learning and teaching

Patient–centred nursing care

In the latter part of the previous chapter the preferred approach to the delivery of professional nursing care was identified as the use of the nursing process. The nursing process as a work method and its potential scientific, logical and rational aspects were also explored. The development of abilities and skills in problem–solving learning were compared to those required for use of the nursing process. However, in the literature reviewed there was only limited evidence that teaching and learning of problem–solving in a classroom context results in development of critical thinking skills as required for nursing practice. Furthermore Tanner (1990) claims that the rational–technical epistemiology of practice is the mere application of scientific knowledge to technical problem–solving and the assumptions of this epistemiology cannot hold up in the complex and uncertain field of professional practice. For example, regard is not taken of the complex and unique nature of people.

The unique nature of people is addressed in humanistic philosophy. It can be shown also in the published literature that values and beliefs embedded both in student–centred learning and teaching and the nursing process stem broadly from humanistic philosophy. For example, Carter (1979) and Webb (1979) identify that a patient–centred philosophy as exampled in the use of the nursing process is underpinned by humanistic philosophy. Likewise Joseph (1985) identifies that student–centred education has very similar philosophical underpinnings. Therefore in the following section of this literature review the dimensions of humanistic values and the nursing process and patient–centred care will be explored.

Humanism

King and Gerwig (1981) describe a humanistic orientation as that which sees people as 'unified wholes' and as active beings who search for meaning in their lives. A person in this philosophy is more than the sum of their parts: each has personal and unique needs, desires, fears and abilities.

Joseph (1985) examines the tenets of humanism in more detail and drawing upon the work of Burber (1967), Sarton (1937), Sartre (1977) and Zahorik and Brubaker (1972), identifies them as the following:

1 Adherence to a naturalistic view of the world.
2 Beliefs in the unity of body and soul.
3 All problems can solved by research and the application of the scientific method.
4 Individuals are responsible for making their own choices and are accountable for their actions.
5 People have a value and worth and strive to meet their maximum potential.

Joseph concludes that as a philosophy humanism can easily incorporate compatible values about clients, students and nursing education. Central to these values are views of personhood.

Personhood

Compatibility between patient–centred nursing and educational perspectives on student–centred learning with regard to personhood can be demonstrated from views expressed in the literature. For example, Carter (1979) and Webb (1979) state that beliefs about personhood are focal features of the nursing process, and views of personhood in an educational context are explored by Jarvis (1986). Jarvis considers that, whilst the type of learner in the educational process is important whether it be child or adult, of more crucial importance is that education is viewed as a process that concerns people irrespective of their age. Education of equals is said to concentrate upon the person and educational processes on the nature and development of the person.

Alternative perspectives to these views of personhood are, however, investigated by Henry and Tuxill (1987). The biological or reductionist view of person is explored and identified to be a hall–mark of traditional approaches to nursing practice. This traditional approach is seen as being incompatible with the humanistic philosophy of the nursing process and of student–centred learning. For example, a reductionist nursing perspective views patients as merely biologically dysfunctioning or potentially dysfunctioning beings and therefore ignores the holistic features of humanistic philosophy which sees the person in a unified or holistic way. However, whilst biological reductionism is not an explicit aspect of the philosophy of the nursing process, an arguably implicit feature is that of its logical rational view of personhood.

Views of personhood and patients are proposed by a number of nurse theorists with regard to conceptual models of nursing care. For example, Henderson (1966) claims that the human mind and body are inseparable and concepts of persons should include biological, psychological, sociological and spiritual components. Orem (1980) views people as seeking self–care and nursing as focussing on human beings. Roy (1976) regards the person as a holistic adaptive system. Neuman (1982) also emphasizes a whole–person concept but in a systems approach identifies variables that may affect human life. Finally Peplau (1952) in a developmental model emphasizes personal growth of both nurse and patient and sees all individuals as unique people with both biological and psychological components who are capable of achieving new learning and making positive changes.

It is clear that all these conceptual views of the person given in a nursing framework have differing emphasis on the nature of personhood. Pearson and Vaughan (1990) state that this is reflected in the appropriate use of different care models in different care settings. One central flaw in many of these theories of nursing is, however, identified by Taylor (1992) and this is that nurses as people are absent from a great many of the theories. It is therefore under–recognised that patients and nurses share a common humanity. However, it is evident that, with regard to patients as people, all have similar humanistic underpinnings albeit with differing emphases.

Individualised patient care

Wilson–Barnett (1988) in the United Kingdom examines recent popular cliches inherent in nursing values. The concept of individualised, holistic or patient–centred care is identified as being one of the most commonly currently used cliches in nursing. However, the research evidence reviewed by Wilson–Barnett would vindicate this as not just a cliche but a practised value.

Sheahan (1982) in a study conducted in the United Kingdom found that when students enter nursing they are person–centred. Rolfe (1993b) also, when developing a scale to measure patient–centredness in student nurses, found that only 16 pre–registration student nurses out of a sample of 327 from 5 colleges of nursing had scores which fell within the noticeably untherapeutic level. However, as the students in these studies were in their first few weeks of training, the findings may be seen rather to validate the need for appropriate selection procedures for training, than to evaluate the effectiveness of educational programmes in imparting the importance of patient–centred care.

Attitudes of student nurses to patient–centred care were also examined by Burnard and Morrison (1991). However, this study was conducted at a later point in training than those previously described. The focus of the study was counselling skills, and attitudes of a group of qualified and student nurses to client–centred care were examined. It was found that students were more client–centred than were trained nurses.

Other authors, however, contest the view that patient–centredness is a consistent feature of nursing practice. For example, in a North American context, Fenton (1986) reports that there is a lack of evidence that practising nurses consistently incorporate the values of humanism in their roles and give individualised care. It is concluded from the evidence of the studies reviewed by Fenton that, although nursing has described itself as humanistic, it is not an approach routinely occurring in hospital settings. Bradham et al (1990) also in a North American study, however, explores the wider dimension of desirable nursing attributes. A profile of personality traits desirable for nurses was developed from a survey of 178 Registered Nurses studying at 4 different institutions. The scores for the valued traits were then compared to the scores of a second sample of student nurses (n=90). It was found that there was some divergence of opinion between the two groups, however, there was strong agreement to the nurturance category. Both groups laid emphasis on the nurturing, comforting or caring role of nurses.

Care and care–giving

More recent developments in individualised nursing have had the concept of care as a central feature. For example, the essence of nursing practice is described by a number of authors as that of care and care–giving (Darbyshire 1991, Farmer 1992, McFarlane 1976, Morse et al 1990, Tanner 1990). However, care as a concept in nursing practice is identified by Morrison (1991) as multi–faceted. The whole gamut of the nursing role and function is incorporated into the construct analysis Morrison gives. However, physical care–giving and the emotional aspects of care are two of the broad dimensions of care he describes.

The emotional, loving dimension of care–giving has been contrasted to a scientific construct (which may be compared to the rational logical view of personhood given earlier) and has been examined by a number of other authors (Arndt 1992, Chipman 1991, Jacono 1993, Komorita et al 1991, Mallik 1988, Mangold 1991, May 1991, Morrison 1991, Schroeder and Neil 1992, Smith 1991, Sprengel and Kelley 1992). Feminist critiques of the ethics of caring and social expectations of females as care–givers have also been addressed in the literature reviewed (Condon 1992, Gordon 1991). However, Griffin (1983) sees care in a wider dimension as a moral recognition of the status of patients as persons and as equitable to the holistic values inherent in patient–centred care.

Other affective qualities of nursing practice have also been examined, for example, the concept of trust by Meize–Grochowski (1984) and Thorne and Robinson (1988), and empathy by Reynolds and Presly (1988). However, in patients' views the relative important of these affective qualities of nursing may be seen to be at variance with dominant nursing values. For example, Darbyshire (1991) states that the educational emphasis in nurse training should not be on technical competence but on compassion and caring. However, Komorita et al (1991) and Larson (1984) found that competent technical know–how was ranked very high by the patients surveyed. This differed from the nurses studied, who regarded psychosocial skills as indicative of caring behaviour. Cronin and Harrison (1988) did a qualitative study and came to similar conclusions to Komorita and Larson, namely that behaviours perceived as caring by patients focused on technical competence. Patients believed that certain minimum requirements such as cleanliness and feeding must be met before more qualitative aspects of care, such as empathy, could be addressed.

It may be concluded from this section and previous sections of this literature review that the individual person is the central character for concern whether in student–centred education or patient–centred care. However, in both settings there is conflicting evidence as to whether or not these values are incorporated into either in nursing or educational practices. However, clearly of pivotal importance in both the delivery of nursing care using a patient–centred approach and the learning and teaching continuum are the nature of person and person to person interactions.

Student nurse/nurse teacher and student nurse/patient relationships

It was shown in the previous chapter that generally effectiveness of manifestations of student–centred learning in nursing could not be verified using published research findings. However, the focus of that part of the review was mainly on classroom teaching and learning methods and expectations of student nurse roles. In the following section the importance of student/teacher relationships and roles of nurse teachers will be of central concern.

Role limitation

An area not explored previously is that of role imitation, or whether the behaviour characteristics displayed by nurse teachers are imitated and mirrored in student nurse/patient relationships. The basic question addressed is whether student–centred teaching and learning principles adopted by nurse teachers in providing educational experiences are imitated by student nurses and used as a basis for role modelling in patient care delivery.

Bandura (1977) proposes that the fundamental means by which new modes of behaviour are acquired involves imitation or observational learning. Social learning therefore involves the acquisition of those behaviour patterns which society or a profession expects. Bandura also believes that self–efficacy, or the degree of confidence in our ability to behave in a socially skilled way, is dependent on prolonged exposure to a graded model, the provision of reinforcement by a competent supervisor, and a situation where anxiety is kept to a minimum. It is therefore possible that students' self–efficacy may be positively influenced by continual presence of a competent, non–threatening role model.

A number of authors hypothesise that there are inter–relationships between the way nursing students are taught and the way they care for patients (Beckett and Wall 1985, Betz 1985, Carter 1978, Clarridge et al 1992, Mander 1992, Nelms et al 1993, Reynolds and Presly 1988). The structured use of role modelling of caring scenarios by teachers has also been investigated by a number of nurse researchers. For example, Lopez (1983) and Nelms et al (1993) in North America found that students responded positively and learnt caring behaviour from faculty role–modelling. However, caring was also learned from other health care staff encountered and it was found that caring can be learned from non–caring behaviour. In the United Kingdom Hodges (1991) conducted an experimental study with two groups of student nurses (n=26). Role modelling the constructs of empathy was compared to theoretical teaching sessions. Data obtained from Patient Interview Assessment Schedules revealed no differences between the groups in relation to increasing interactive empathy.

It may be concluded that the learning effectiveness of role-modelling or role-play as a teaching method cannot be verified from the published research. However, no published research findings have been uncovered in the course of this literature search into the part role imitation plays in learning appropriate care delivery behaviour.

Effective teaching behaviour

Definitions of effective teaching behaviour have been the focus of a number of studies in North America. For example, Eason and Corbett (1991) in a survey of 2877 qualified nurses identified 20 desirable attributes of nurse teachers which had a ranking frequency of 5 or more. Being helpful, informative and interesting were the highest ranking attributes. Schumann (1990) analysed post registration course evaluations (n=405). The quality of teaching was found to be a focal issue. Positive teaching attributes were identified as being assertive, self–assured, empathetic, accepting of students, non–judgemental, trustworthy, sincere, sensitive, competent, knowledgeable, honest, democratic, supportive, and resourceful.

Sheahan (1981), however, in a survey in the United Kingdom examined how nurse tutors (93) and student nurses (n=317) perceive the role of nurse teacher. It was found there was only agreement between the two groups on four of twelve factors. The students in the study were found to emphasise the importance of the moral/pastoral roles of teachers and also wanted teachers to be clinical specialists. However, there was agreement on teachers being role models to learn from and of the importance of student–centred learning.

Alderton (1983), Baker (1982), Davidson (1992), Farabaugh (1984), Lindop (1991), Pugh (1986) and Rice (1992), however, give views of the nursing educational process from a student nurses' perspective. Many accounts are critical of clinical experiences. For example, Davidson reports that she left nursing because she had been unable to care for patients in the ways taught in the classroom. Lindop, also in a study of why nurses leave training, found unsatisfactory clinical experiences to be a major reason. Farabaugh and Pugh give similar viewpoints but criticise nurse teachers for not preparing students for the realities of care settings.

The research evidence can be seen to give some validity to these mainly anecdotal accounts. For example, Rachal and DeCoux (1992) in North America investigated the teaching behaviours of post–graduate student adult educators (n=90). It was found that the nurse educators had a more pedagogical orientation than did the general population of adult educators.

Theis (1988) also in a North American study looked at the dimensions of respect and justice as typified in nurse teachers' behaviour. It was found, in a sample of senior nursing students (n=204) from 3 baccalaureate programmes, that 167 respondents reported a total of 216 examples of unethical teaching behaviour. Baxter (1992) also found evidence of nurse teachers labelling as trouble–makers students who challenged the existing order.

Davies (1991), similarly in a study of change at a nurse educational institute in the United Kingdom, found a perceived gulf in the educational hierarchy. In a sample of students, teachers and educational managers (n=67), whilst good change scenarios were identified as being dependent on open trusting relationships, in reality such relationships were not found to exist.

Contrary to these finding Davies (1984) in the United Kingdom, when conducting an ethnographic study of student nurses (n=24) attitudes from 4 schools of nursing, found that comments about the school and tutors had the highest frequencies. Two thirds were positive with regard to the support and guidance they received from their teachers. Negative and positive comments of ward staff were, however, more equally divided.

It may be concluded on balance from the albeit limited findings of these studies that student nurses are generally critical of their learning experiences. Ineffective teaching behaviours obviously may have detrimental effects on learning outcomes and the patient care given by these student nurses. However, the effects of teaching can be seen to be not only of importance in terms of achieving learning outcomes but in the influence it has on individual students' self–concepts and self–worth. Therefore teaching behaviour and student nurses' self–concept will be examined in the following section of this chapter.

Teaching behaviour and students nurses' self–concepts

During occupational socialisation student nurses acquire a concept of self as a nurse. Some educational processes have been shown to have a detrimental effect on aspects of self–concept. The realities of clinical experience and negative teaching qualities have been shown previously to be major factors which may impinge students' self–concepts.

Hammer and Tufts 1985 describe how nurse educators can foster a positive self–image in their students. Various teaching strategies are suggested, the use of which it is suggested may enhance student nurses' self–concepts. However, Hammer and Tufts offer no evaluation regarding their use.

In North American Ellis's (1980) findings, in a similar vein to previously reviewed studies, also show that senior nursing students in clinical areas lacked self–confidence. and Ellis proposed that nurse teachers contributed to this self–destruction of self–concept by the teaching methods used. Klug (1989) also observed a negative change in self–concept over a 2 year period amongst baccalaureate students. Likewise Cotanch (1981) found in a sample 498 nursing students at 2 universities that self–actualising scores were higher in the more junior students. However, Shepherd and Brookes (1991) examined differences between diploma, associate degree and baccalaureate student nurses' self–concepts. Mean scores for all groups fell within the realms of satisfactory self–concept for all the groups. Ellis (1980), contrary to the findings of Cotanch, found in a sample (n=177) of nursing students that self–confidence and self–esteem were low at the beginning of course and high at its conclusion

Studies in North America have also investigated other factors which may affect students' self–esteem. For example, Hilbert and Allen (1985) hypothesized that there would be a positive relationship between high levels of social and family support and self–esteem in nursing students. However, in a study at one university using a sample junior (n=67) and senior (n=60) nursing students there was found to be no such correlation.

In the United Kingdom Champion (1991) also reports that raising self–esteem of students is crucial in the teaching process. However, Taylor (1993) observes that it would seem that current educational processes in nursing are designed to keep students from knowing themselves or their nursing environment in any realistic way. Studies into self–concept in the United Kingdom confirm conclusions drawn at earlier points in the literature review. For example, in an ethnographic study Neal (1989) found that it was the students with a low self–esteem who could not handle realities of patient care. Bradby's (1990) study, which used as a sample 4 cohorts from 2 schools of nursing, also shows that the status transition into the occupational role of the nurse is easier for those who have higher self–esteem and lower anxiety scores.

Gates (1989) investigated teacher behaviour and its effects on nursing students' self–esteem. It was found that measures of teaching behaviour were difficult to quantify and therefore there was insufficient experimental manipulation of the independent variable to extrapolate meaningful interpretation. There were, however, no significant of differences in the students' self–esteem as measured before and after experimental teaching sessions.

It can be concluded from these studies that there is conflicting evidence with regard to the effects of nurse educational programmes on student nurses' self–concepts. Relationships between self–concept and confidence in clinical experiences, however, appear to be integrally linked.

Power and control in teacher/student/patient relationships

Dufault (1985) describes how distribution of power and control in teacher/student relationships is also associated with self–esteem. Self–responsible and self–directed practitioners are seen as having an internal locus of control which in turn, it is hypothesised by Dufault, leads to high self–esteem. This may be compared to an external locus of control of, for example, a teacher located power base, which Dufault believes is associated with poor self–esteem, depression and 'burn out'.

Dufault (1985) in North America conducted a study which had as its focus evaluation of a futuristic–oriented seminar course. The course focused on the skills and knowledge needed for life–long professional development. A sample 64 Registered Nurses and the Rotter Internal–External Locus of Control Scale were used. It was found that pre– and post–course test scores for the experimental group and control group were significantly different. The experimental group demonstrated a significantly higher scores on an internal locus of control.

Brown (1993) in the United Kingdom, using a qualitative approach examined nurse teachers' (n=4) and student nurses' (n=5) perceptions of power in their relationships. The evidence suggested that the teachers wished to be power sharers. However, the students' primary concern was for an effective interpersonal relationship with their nurse teachers. Approachability/ disclosure/respect mechanisms described by the students in this study are congruent with Rogers' (1983) 'freedom to learn model'

Similar concepts of empowerment can be seen to feature in models of nursing care. For example, the previously described model of Orem's (1980) has self–care as a major emphasis. The central belief in this model is that the nursing function should be directed to enable and allow people to take the initiative in being responsible for their own health care when this is possible. Norris (1979) suggests that as an idea self–care arose in consumer groups in the 1960s, beginning with anti–professional and anti–intellectual feelings and an urge to return to the kind of life which emphasises 'being human'.

Kasch (1986) also believes that effecting positive changes in patients' health status depends on nurse–patient interactions that promote consensus. Consensus is arrived at through the process of negotiation. However, successful outcomes depend on the nurse's interpersonal skills. Morse (1991) similarily describes that a successful nurse–patient relationship is the result of covert negotiations. Distortions of the ideal relationship are said to occur if the nurse is unwilling or unable to be committed to the patient. The patient will in response use manipulative or coercive behaviours in an attempt to increase nursing involvement in the relationship. If patients are unwilling to trust the nurse or accept their illness situation, they will manifest 'difficult' behaviours, be withdrawn, or try to escape altogether from the relationship.

Malin and Teasdale (1991), however, argue that there is an inherent tension between the concepts of caring and empowerment. For example, a nurse adopts a caring role when doing things for patients or when protecting them from harm or unnecessary worry. The power base is not equal in this situation but may be likened to that between a child and parent. Malin and Teasdale identify that a central question nursing needs to address is the tension between empowerment and caring as central values. Consideration also is needed of the extent to which patients actually wish to become partners in nurse/patient relationships.

In the following chapter the general conclusions that may be drawn from this literature review will be considered. The research questions stemming from these conclusions will also be identified.

4 Conclusions drawn from the literature review and the research questions

In previous chapters it has been shown that how student–centred learning and teaching is defined is seen as being contentious and confused with concepts inherent in andragogical tenets, in the perspectives of the majority of authors writing in a nurse educational context. For example, the term student–centred learning was shown to be often used in a practical sense of how nurse education should be conducted, whereas the term andragogy was used to denote a value–system underpinning the practicalities of nurse education.

That student–centred learning and teaching and andragogy are currently favoured in nursing educational philosophies may be demonstrated by the abundance of literature reviewed. However, the conclusion drawn from the review of the literature is that there is little evidence that demonstrates how deeply embedded these beliefs are in nurse education value systems. Also there is little evidence that these beliefs influence how nurse education is articulated in teaching and learning processes.

How these general conclusions are drawn is the focus of the following section of this study when the way the literature review was conducted is examined.

Conducting the literature search

In the initial phrase of the literature search the broad headings of student–centred learning and patient–centred care were used as key words. However, in regard to student–centred learning only a limited amount of pertinent literature was found. It was evident that a wider focus other than student–centred learning was required. Through analysis of published works andragogy was identified as an important concept. However, again there was only a limited amount of published material that covered andragogical concepts in their broader manifestations. In addition literature obtained was exhortative and anecdotal in nature. There were, for example, extremely few articles which based opinions on either student–centred learning and teaching or andragogical theories in nurse education on empirical findings.

The final phase of exploration of the literature related to student–centred learning and teaching involved using discrete topics. These topics corresponded to the broad tenets of student–centred learning and andragogy identified in the initial phases of the literature review. Major influences in identifying these topics were the work of cognitivists such as Bruner (1966) and exponents of andragogy such as Knowles (1980). The discrete topics were self–directed, experiential and problem–solving learning. The subsequent search of the literature pertaining to these topics revealed a substantial amount of published work. Management of the large amounts of literature eventually acquired was therefore to a certain extent simplified by taking this approach. For example, the major categories of student–centred learning and teaching and andragogical concepts were the starting point of the literature search. Subsequent categories were developed from identification of the three discrete areas of student–centred learning, namely those of self–directed, experiential and problem–solving learning. Sub–categories of these three areas were also developed. For example, reflective learning became a sub–group of experiential teaching and learning. A coded index system was utilised to record salient features of the literature reviewed.

The second stage of the literature search had patient–centred care as a focus. It was demonstrated in chapter 3 that an abundance of literature was obtained relating to the nursing process as a system of care delivery. There were numerous descriptive and evaluative studies which centred on use of the nursing process. Patient–centred nursing care, humanism, personhood and individualised patient care were identified as key concepts. Key concepts of student–centred learning and teaching were identified as effective teaching behaviours, the development of self–concept and power and control. Care and care–giving were identified as unifying concepts. However, when literature was sought which compared and contrasted nurse/client/patient relationships to student nurse/nurse teacher relationships, in a care and care–giving context, there was very little. Whilst a number of authors identified the possibility of bridging the theory:practice gap in nurse education through student nurses role modelling appropriate teacher caring–giving behaviour no research evidence was uncovered which verified this hypothesis.

Analysis of the findings of the literature review

Analysis of the findings of literature reviewed in chapters 2 and 3 illustrates that articulation of student–centred learning and teaching principles in the delivery of nurse education is a complex subject area. The literature reviewed demonstrates that there has been very limited research conducted into the subject area. There have, for example, been no large scale research projects which examine the efficacy of student–centred learning methods in nurse education. Also little replicated research has been conducted. Generally the research reviewed gives a fragmented picture with little evidence of a research base underpinning current practices in nurse education. For example, evaluation of the albeit limited research into application of student–centred learning and teaching in nursing education gives conflicting evidence. It cannot be shown that use of any of the approaches to teaching and learning is completely validated. Indeed the majority of evidence does not support the effectiveness of student–centred learning and teaching principles.

Views on the effectiveness of student–centred learning and teaching can be seen also to differ between those teaching and those being taught. Whilst values of autonomy and independence are a focal feature of student–centred learning and teaching, these principles cannot be seen to be evident in their practical application. Indeed there is limited evidence that although student–centred approaches are being deployed by nurse teachers this is without consultation with students being taught. Differences can also be identified in views on the importance of teaching and learning environments. Emphasis in the literature review has been mainly on classroom teaching and learning. Nursing students can, however, be seen to view clinical experience as the most valuable form of learning experience.

The need for classroom teaching in pre–registration nurse training courses is clear. A pre–registration training system which is purely clinically based is clearly not an educationally sound approach and is incompatible with service priorities for care delivery. Learning nursing by a 'sitting by Nelly' approach or an apprenticeship–type system has been demonstrated in the past to be an ineffective and at times dangerous approach (Baly 1980, Dingwall et al 1988). However, effectiveness of classroom teaching and the balance and integration of classroom teaching with clinical teaching can be identified as being problematic. The theory:practice divide in nurse education is a subject which nurse educationists still need to address.

In the latter part of the literature review the preferred approach to the delivery of patient care was identified as use of the nursing process. Patient–centred care as epitomised in this method of nursing was shown as having similar philosophical roots to student–centred learning, namely humanism. However, there is little evidence that a philosophy of humanism as embedded in the ideals of patient–centred care are featured in the reality of care–giving.

Identified also in the literature reviewed was the potential tension between humanistic philosophy and concepts of the person in a rational, logical perspective typified in a nursing process approach. However, this tension was shown to have been partially counter–balanced by recent interest in the affective qualities of care–giving. It was also identified that emphasis on the comforting, compassionate and empathic dimensions of care has been criticised by some. For example, there is a possible incompatibility of these values, and the needs and values of patients. In the literature reviewed patients were shown to value more highly technical nursing competencies than the affective aspects of care–giving.

Of central concern in the literature review was the nature of student nurse/teacher relationships and how this may be reflected and mirrored in student nurse/patient relationships. Social learning theory was identified as a theory which gives a comprehensive explanation of the phenomenon of role–imitation. The dimensions of effective teaching and teaching behaviour were also explored in the context of effects on student nurses' self–concept. Power and control were identified as having a pivotal effect on both students' and patients' self–concepts. However, it was shown that patients may be more accepting of unequal power relationships and passivity in nurse/patient relationships than are student nurses in student nurse/nurse teacher relationships.

Whilst critiques of the research studies reviewed have been given in the previous chapters, it can be summarised that any conclusions drawn are based on very limited empirical research evidence which stems from studies conducted mainly in North America. Much of this research can be seen to comply with positivistic–type research principles. Also the often small sample sizes and difficulties with accurate measurement call into question how reliable and valid are the findings of many of the studies reviewed. In comparison there has been even more limited research conducted in the United Kingdom. However, this research is not dominated by a single research philosophy. Approximately equal examples of interpretative and positivistic research frameworks have been found in the United Kingdom studies. Nevertheless there are similar reliability and validity issues as with the North American studies.

Research questions

There are a number of broad areas which can be identified as arising out of the literature review which warrant further investigation. There are for example general questions relating to the conundrum of what student–centred learning and teaching and andragogy are taken to mean by nurse educators. There are also more specific questions about the effectiveness of student–centred learning and teaching methods as used in nurse education. There are also general questions in respect of relationships between how student nurses are taught and how they approach patient care. More specific questions relate to what part nurse teachers play in the process of student nurses' learning to care.

The research questions which stem from this literature review are therefore as follows:

1. What are the attitudes of senior nurse education managers in institutions where pre–registration nurse training occurs regarding the concepts of andragogy and student–centred learning and teaching?
2. What are the values and perceptions of nurse teachers regarding the concepts of andragogy and student–centred learning and teaching and patient–centred nursing care?
3. What are the values and perceptions of pre–registration student nurses regarding the concepts of student–centred learning and teaching?
4. How do pre–registration student nurses' Patient–Centred Multi–Choice Questionnaire (PMQX) scores compare to their institutions' Student–Centred Learning and Teaching Attitude Questionnaire (SAQ) scores?

The research questions are specifically focused in terms of both subject areas and sample groupings. This has been done to keep the study manageable and compatible with researcher resources.

5 Research methods

In the previous chapter a number of research questions which stemmed from the review of the literature were identified. The aim of this chapter is to describe the research design used to explore these research questions and to discuss methodological issues.

Methodological issues

Nisbet and Entwhistle (1974) define educational research as:

> a careful and systematic attempt to understand the educational process and, through understanding to improve the system. (p.7)

The purpose of this study is to explore relationships between the ways pre-registration student nurses are taught about nursing and attitudes to care delivery using a survey approach. Nisbet and Entwhistle's definition is therefore of particular relevance to this investigation as information generated may give a clearer picture of opinions of how pre-registration student nurses should be taught, the actuality of how they are taught, and whether it is perceived that there are any interconnections between approaches to teaching and learning and approaches to the delivery of patient care. The investigation will therefore have a utilitarian value for improving patient care.

Sheenan (1986) describes research methodology as the:

> description and analysis of research methods which throws light on their limitations and resources and clarifies their presuppositions and consequencies. (p.196)

Research methodology issues therefore address problems that are inherent in the use of particular strategies of collecting data. There are issues surrounding measurement and the research tools' reliability, or the dependability with which an instrument measures the attribute it is designed to measure. There are also issues of validity or the degree to which an instrument measures what it is intended to be measured. Issues concerning advantages and disadvantages of the research methods used or their reliability will be highlighted in the following description of the research approaches. Issues pertaining to research validity will also be discussed.

Student-centred attitude questionnaire (SAQ)

A number of differing research approaches are used in the study, including methods which fall into the general remit of experimental research with its underpinning philosophy of positivism. For example, there is an attempt to apply scientific principles to collection and analysis of data. Also included are methods which belong to a broadly interpretative approach. There is therefore an aim to collect data which are both qualitative and quantitative in nature.

Attitude analysis

Of central concern in the first part of the study is attitude analysis or the general values held within nurse education in England regarding approaches to teaching and learning in pre-registration nurse education. For example, the first research question addresses the attitudes of those in positions of influence in nurse education regarding student-centred learning and teaching and andragogy. The question also addresses the lack of research evidence regarding dominant value systems of learning and teaching philosophies in pre-registration nurse education in England.

Shaw and Wright (1977) describe how use and definition of the term attitude varies. The psychological construct of attitude, however, views an attitude as an end product of socialisation processes which significantly influences the person's responses to others or groups of others. Attitude is thus viewed as a learned response which has been developed through the influence of the multitude of variables involved in socialisation processes.

Anderson and Fishbein (1965) define attitude as an evaluative response or strength of beliefs about given topic or situation. There is therefore in social interaction a pre-disposition to respond in certain ways. However, Cardno (1955) cautions that such responses are not only the result of previous learning responses but are also influenced by an individual's perception and interpretation of the current social circumstances. In other words, measurement of attitudes will only identify a predisposition for behaviour and will not be a reliable predictor of future behaviour. Such future behaviour is determined by an interaction of previously learned attitudes and individual's evaluation of current social circumstances.

Measurement of attitudes

Pennington (1986) describes two differing approaches to discovery of what people's attitudes are to a given topic or situation. These are those of indirect and direct measures. Indirect measures include physiological techniques, such as, for example, galvanic skin responses, heart rate or pupillary dilation. However, Pennington goes on to state that there is little evidence that shows a correlation between such measures and attitude.

The use of attitude or rating scales as a direct measure of attitudes is described by Shaver (1986). Shaver identifies four major techniques: Priori scaling, Thurstone scaling, Likert scaling and semantic differential scaling.

Priori scales are described by Shaver (1986) as the crudest method of measuring attitudes. The scales consist of a case study method or questions on a specific topic area followed by ballot counting of agreement or disagreement answers. They are therefore in effect 2 point scales and only measure extremes of attitudes.

A Thurstone scale is comprised of a number of items to which respondents are invited to give a graded response within a strong agreement to strong disagreement range. Compiling such a scale consists briefly of surveying a large sample opinions to a given topic area. These opinion statements are given to large group of judges with instructions to sort opinion statements into 11 piles - an 11 point scale. Distributions are tabulated for each statement which form the criteria for constructing the scale. The scale is built up by choosing a number of items which have low distribution values.

The Likert scale is a modification of the Thurstone scale and makes assumptions that attitudes are distributed normally. Such scales measure attitudes using standard deviation units. Between scale values are obtained by this method and numerical values from, for example, 1 to 5 are assigned to responses.

A semantic differential scale also provides a pre-selected series of statements to which respondents are asked to agree or disagree as does the Thurstone scale. However, it also gives a 7-point bipolar adjective scale on which concepts are judged. It provides, as Shaver (1986) describes, three-dimensional information: negative or positive feelings, potency or strength of feelings and significance of opinions to respondents.

A literature search for a scale of any type failed to reveal the existence of one suitable for use in this study, and therefore the attitude scale used in the first part of this study has been developed by the researcher.

Development of the attitude questionnaire

A number of methodological problems may be identified with each of the scales described earlier. Identification and exploration of these problems influenced construction of the scale used in this study. Whilst a Priori scale would be simple to compile, would be an extremely crude measure of attitudes. Complexity of compiling a Thurstone or semantic scale was seen as being unrealistic in terms of resources available. The choice of scale for use of the study is therefore a 5 point Likert scale.

Items of the rating scale used in this investigation were selected on the basis of major themes identified by the literature search. Therefore various sections of the literature review are mirrored in the items given in the scale. It is argued that by taking this approach an element of consensus of expert opinion is incorporated into the basic framework of the scale, the expert opinion being authors of literature reviewed.

It should, however, be noted that as the attitude questionnaire is developed from the relevant literature examined prior to conducting the research, therefore the literature review given in chapters 2 and 3 has not been amended or updated. It is believed that the literature reviewed prior to conducting the research is an integral feature of the attitude questionnaire design and therefore should be examined as such. However, there is an intention to compare the results of the study with relevant published findings. Therefore additional current literature will be included in the chapter devoted to discussion of the findings of the study.

The basic framework of the scale was devised to address two discrete areas identified in the literature review. The first of these areas pertained to attitudes regarding dimensions of student-centred teaching and learning in nurse education. So, for example, do nurse educators see student-centredness as being comprised of an andragogical approach which develops self-directed learning skills, incorporates active learning methodologies and problem-solving activities? The second area addresses whether it is felt that principles of student-centred teaching and learning are used in pre-registration nurse education in the various institutions surveyed. For example, is it believed that andragogical approaches and dimensions of student-centred learning and teaching are used in the respondent's educational institution during pre-registration training?

The devised attitude statements were incorporated into a questionnaire to which was added questions regarding biographical details. Included were respondent details, types of pre-registration courses offered, student intake numbers and taught class size. These variables were selected to allow analysis of differences between, for example, differing types of pre-registration courses. Class size was seen as an important variable in terms of acting as potential constraint to uses of student-centred learning and teaching methods. A concluding question was added which asked if respondents would be willing to participate further in the study.

There was an intention throughout the design phase of the questionnaire to keep it relatively simple and short. A self-return postal survey was envisaged, and therefore the time taken to complete the questionnaire would be factor that could influence the return rate. A 15 minute completion time was the aim. By doing this it was hoped that an optimum return rate would be achieved. Also in the wider context of the study the attitude survey was seen as only providing a general picture. At later points of the investigation use of indepth qualitative research methods would give more detailed data.

Pilot study of the attitude questionnaire

The SAQ was designed to be distributed to principals of colleges of nursing and heads of departments in higher educational institutions. Therefore initial phases of the pilot study involved interviews with two principals of colleges of nursing and one head of department of a higher education institution.

From the findings of the interviews a number of changes were identified as necessary. Main areas of change were to the biographical part of the questionnaire. These changes related to clarifying the exact nature of student groups the study was focussing on. For example, it was seen as being necessary to clearly state that midwifery, second registration and conversion students were not included in the survey. Phrasing of questions related to student intake numbers was also seen as unclear. For example, one principal said it would be unrealistic to give a prediction of student intake numbers as regional contracts for nurse education were done on a year to year basis. Therefore the question was re-phrased to relate only to current student cohort sizes.

A further point made by one of the principals was that it would be unlikely that they would complete the questionnaire themselves, but would give it to a member of staff who had direct responsibility for pre-registration training. Therefore a further three interviews were conducted with course directors of pre-registration nurse education. A question was also added to the questionnaire relating to the respondent's position in the education establishment.

The second series of interviews was conducted in a similar fashion to the first. The subjects were individuals the principals and head of department identified as being most likely to be asked to complete the questionnaire. Changes that were identified as being necessary by these interviewees were to questions in the biographical section which related to class size. This was seen by the interviewees as being likely to be very different in a Common Foundation Course to Branch programmes and between differing Branch programmes. Therefore further questions were added to this section.

Two interviewees also commented that items on the rating scale seemed very biased towards obtaining positive responses. This comment was similar to one made by the head of department in the first series of interviews. Therefore three questions on beliefs regarding dimensions of student-centred learning were changed to a negative direction. Similarly three questions regarding whether or not student-centred learning is practised in the respondent's educational institution were also changed to a negative direction.

The final part of the pilot study was aimed to estimate the reliability of the SAQ. The sample used in this part of the pilot study was two groups of nurse teacher students (n=22). This convenience sample was seen to be matched on a number of variables. They were, for example, of similar ages, sex and occupation. Respondents were also undertaking similar study modules, that is educational theory and curriculum studies, albeit at differing education levels.

The respondents were asked to complete the questionnaire when attending a lesson taught by the researcher. It was stated that completion of the questionnaire was entirely optional and respondents were assured of anonymity. However, all the student teachers present did agree to take part in the study which may indicate a wish to be compliant to the wishes of the researcher rather than a true desire to participate in the study.

Data obtained from this part of the pilot study was coded for statistical analysis utilising SPSSX. Table 5.1 gives the general statistical analysis of the data.

Table 5.1

Frequencies, means, modes, ranges and standard deviations of the pilot study attitude questionnaire

	Value	Freq	Mean	Median	Range	S.D.
Att 1	1	11	2.136	1	4.000	1.390
	2	4				
	3	1				
	4	5				
	5	1				
Att 2	1	0	3.682	4	3.000	.894
	2	3				
	3	4				
	4	12				
	5	3				
Att 3	1	9	2.000	2	3.000	1.069
	2	7				
	3	3				
	4	3				
	5	0				
Att 4	1	9	1.682	2	3.000	.716
	2	12				
	3	1				
	4	0				
	5	0				
Att 5	1	7	2.273	2	3.000	1.077
	2	5				
	3	7				
	4	3				
	5	0				
Att 6	1	3	3.227	3	4.000	1.232
	2	2				
	3	7				
	4	7				
	5	3				
Att 7	1	0	3.445	3	3.000	.963
	2	4				
	3	7				
	4	8				
	5	3				
Att 8	1	3	2.682	2	4.000	1.211
	2	9				
	3	4				
	4	4				
	5	2				

Table 5.1 cont

Att 9	1 2 3 4 5	8 9 3 2 0	1.955	2	3.000	.950
Att 10	1 2 3 4 5	2 6 5 7 2	3.045	3	4.000	1.174
Att 11	1 2 3 4 5	13 5 3 1 0	1.636	1	3.000	.902
Att 12	1. 2 3 4 5	10 10 0 2 0	1.727	1	3.000	.883
Att 13	1 2 3 4 5	10 5 6 1 0	1.909	2	3.000	.971

The results of the general statistical analysis give an overall picture of agreement with the attitude statements. For example, there are 9 median scores of either strongly agree or agree. In contrast there is only 1 median disagreement score and 3 mid range, neutral responses.

Following general statistical analysis Mann-Whitney analysis was undertaken in order to determine if there were any significant differences between the responses of the two groups. Table 5.2 presents the Mann-Whitney test results. There are no significant differences between the responses of the two groups.

Table 5.2
Mann-Whitney scores of the pilot study SAQ data

	U	2 Tailed Probability
Att 1	49.5	.4770
Att 2	54.5	.6994
Att 3	55.0	.7477
Att 4	58.5	.8977
Att 5	55.0	.7477
Att 6	55.0	.7477
Att 7	50.0	.5190
Att 8	44.5	.3000
Att 9	49.0	.4779
Att 10	42.5	.2426
Att 11	57.0	.8470
Att 12	54.5	.6994
Att 13	39.0	.1713

Table 5.3
Cronbach's alpha scores of the pilot study SAQ data

	Scale mean if item deleted	Scale variance if item deleted	Alpha if item deleted
ATT 1	29.2727	30.9697	.6562
ATT 2	27.7273	35.2554	.6739
ATT 3	29.4091	28.4437	.5873
ATT 4	29.7273	25.5411	.5031
ATT 5	29.1364	25.9329	.5392
ATT 6	28.1818	23.2035	.4911
ATT 7	27.9545	22.9978	.4577
ATT 8	28.7273	27.4459	.5818
ATT 9	29.4545	24.4502	.4943
ATT 10	28.3636	22.2424	.4584
ATT 11	29.7727	23.7078	.4715
ATT 12	29.6818	26.8939	.5435
ATT 13	29.5000	26.8333	.5489

Estimated reliability of the scale 0.6085

The next stage undertaken in measuring the intra-scale reliability of the attitude questionnaire was that of Cronbach Alpha analysis. The Cronbach Alpha results are presented in table 5.3. It can be seen that reliability of some items on the attitude scale is estimated as being less than other items on the scale. Also the overall estimated reliability of 0.6085 can be seen as indicating not a high measure of reliability.

Nunnally (1978), for example, recommends a Cronbach Alpha score of 0.7 and above as giving a reasonable measure of intra-scale reliability. It can be seen that the scores for items 1 and 2 have substantially less reliable scores than the other items. Closer analysis also reveals that these statements relate not to attitude but factual knowledge. Therefore items 1 and 2 were removed from the questionnaire and further Cronbach Alpha analysis undertaken.

Table 5.4 gives the Cronbach Alpha score on the second analysis. A score of 0.7685 can be seen as providing a satisfactory measure of intra-scale reliability.

The final version of the SAQ was distributed as a national survey to educational institutions undertaking pre-registration nurse education in England. The final version of the SAQ is given in Appendix 1.

Table 5.4
Amended Cronbach's alpha scores of the pilot study SAQ data

	Scale mean if item deleted	Scale variance if item deleted	Alpha if item1 and 2 deleted
ATT 3	23.5909	33.4913	.7661
ATT 4	23.9091	30.7532	.7126
ATT 5	23.3182	29.8463	.7246
ATT 6	22.3636	28.3377	.7180
ATT 7	22.1364	27.4567	.6815
ATT 8	22.9091	32.9437	.7712
ATT 9	23.6364	29.1948	.7061
ATT 10	22.5455	27.4026	.6990
ATT 11	23.9545	28.9026	.6986
ATT 12	23.8636	33.2662	.7516
ATT 13	23.6818	31.0844	.7322

Estimated reliability of the scale 0.7685

The SAQ survey

A survey approach is the research methodology used in the first phase of this study. The aim of using this type of methodology is to obtain information regarding the prevalence, distribution and interrelations of attitudes to student-centred learning and teaching and concepts of andragogy in pre-registration nurse education.

The data base for distribution of the SAQ was obtained from the English National Board for Nursing, Midwifery and Health Visiting Applicant Handbook (1993) and Degrees Combined with Nursing and Midwifery Qualifications leaflet (1993). The questionnaire was sent to principals of colleges of nursing in England (n=65) and heads of departments of nursing in higher education institutions (n=25). Returns of the SAQ revealed that two of the colleges of nursing had amalgamated and one higher education institution only offered post-registration education. The final sample was therefore 63 colleges of nursing and 24 institution of higher education (total population 87).

Initial returns of the SAQ gave a response rate of 62% This was seen as being only a moderately good return and therefore a second posting to named individuals was undertaken. Following the second posting a return rate of 87.36% was achieved.

The initial phase of preparing the SAQ data for analysis was that of reverse coding responses to the negatively worded attitude statements so that they were all positively orientated. The attitude survey data was then data coded in regards to the biographical details of the respondents and the characteristics of the educational courses offered by the institutions surveyed. Total mean SAQ scores were also tabulated for each institution.

Difficulties in data coding were, however, identified in regard to reported class size in Common Foundation Programmes. Large differences in estimated class size were reported. Therefore minimum and maximum class sizes were tabulated with estimated ranges of responses. These ranges were then grouped in what was considered to be their major feature. For example, one of these groupings is class size of regularly 30 and under. A response of class size between 10-30 would fall into this grouping. A further example is that of a grouping of class size being reported as on occasions over 100. A response of estimated class size between 15-125 would fall into this grouping. Branch class sizes were, however, omitted from the study as an independent variable because of these difficulties encountered. Appendix 2 gives respondent details.

Data were subsequently analysed using SPSSX. The results of this analysis are presented in the following chapter.

Quantitative versus qualitative research methods

The focus of the first stage of this study was to collect data which is quantitative in nature and to apply 'scientific' principles to its analysis. As described earlier in this chapter there are a number of issues in terms of the validity of research findings that need to be considered. For example, research findings pertaining to attitude analysis cannot be used to predict future behaviour as they are only valid at a given point in time. Therefore attitudes measured by the SAQ instrument are only valid at the time of measurement.

The intention of the second phase of this study is to obtain qualitative data and therefore the type of data collected in the second phase differs to that of the first part of the study. Data collection which has both a qualitative and quantitative is described by Polit and Hungler (1991) as complementary or:

> mutually supplying each other's lack. (p.518)

For example, quantitative data has strengths in terms of generalisability, precision, control over extraneous variables and reliability of measurement but is weak in terms of capturing the intricacies of human beliefs and behaviours. The strengths and weaknesses of quantitative and qualitative methods are therefore complementary, albeit that each stems from very different research traditions. For example, Cowman (1992) considers that qualitative methods develop theory inductively, whilst quantitative research is deductive and its methods are primarily aimed at testing theory.

Traditionally there has been support for the separateness of qualitative and quantitative methods. However, neither method in isolation will providers complete understanding of the intricacies of human beliefs and behaviours. Therefore, whilst the disparate nature of these methods is acknowledged, it is argued that inclusion of both approaches will give deeper and richer insights into the focal issues of this study. Also the validity of the study's findings will be enhanced.

Research triangulation

A further research approach to be incorporated in the study is data triangulation. Denzin (1970) defines triangulation as:

> the combination of multiple methods in a study of the same object or event to depict more accurately the phenomenon being investigated. (p.297)

Denzin (1970) also identifies three basic types of triangulation. These are as follows:

1 Data triangulation which involves collecting data from multiple sources for analysis. Each source is focused upon the phenomenon of interest. There may be three sub-types of data triangulation: time, space and person.
2 Investigator triangulation which concerns use of multiple individuals to collect and analysis a single set of data.
3 Methodological triangulation which involves use of two or more methods of data collection within a single study.

Elements of the majority of these types of triangulation are in part embraced in this study. For example, with regard to data triangulation there is a similar focus of data collection but from a number of different sources and perspectives. Also incorporated is methodological triangulation in the use of multiple methods to collect and analyse the data.

Mitchell (1986) distinguishes between two different forms of methodological triangulation, namely 'within method' and 'across method'. Within method involves use of several different strategies within a single method. An example of this could be using differing scales to measure the same phenomenon. Across method is when dissimilar but complementary methods are used. Across method triangulation is to be utilised in this study. Cowman (1992) relates that a major aim of this method is to achieve convergent validity.

Achieving convergent validity is a central intention of the study design. For example, the initial research focus is to identify how student-centred learning and teaching and concepts of andragogy are articulated in an 'official' sense. This being through identification of attitudes of senior educational managers. These findings will be compared in later stages of the study to both nurse educators' and student nurses' perceptions and beliefs regarding similar topics. An inter-mix of research methods is used at different stages of the study. The second phase of the study, for example, adopts qualitative approach to data collection as compared to the quantitative approach for the SAQ survey.

Nurse teacher interviews

Polit and Hungler (1991) state that qualitative research is based on premises that gaining knowledge about human behaviour is not possible without describing human behaviour as it is lived and defined by the actors themselves. The general aim of the second phase of this study is, therefore, to collect indepth descriptive data which will provide an insightful picture of beliefs and attitudes that nurse teachers hold regarding student-centred learning and teaching and concepts of andragogy.

The approach in the second part of the study consists of conducting a series of focussed interviews with nurse teachers. Aims of these interviews correspond to the second research question given in chapter 3, namely what are the values and perceptions of nurse teachers regarding concepts of student-centred learning and teaching and patient-centred care? New areas of investigation are also introduced. For example, included in the nurse teacher interviews is exploration of the perceived inter-relationships between how pre-registration student nurses are taught and attitudes to care delivery.

The aims of the nurse teacher interviews are therefore designed to address three broad areas. These are as follows:

1 What are nurse teachers' perceptions and beliefs of student-centred learning and teaching and concepts of andragogy?
2 What are nurse teachers' perceptions and beliefs of patient-centred nursing care?
3 Do nurse teachers identify any shared concepts between student-centred learning and teaching and patient-centred nursing care?

The interview schedule devised used these questions as focal areas of enquiry.

Interviews with nurse teachers - pilot study

The sample for the nurse teacher pilot study was selected on the basis of data obtained from the SAQ survey. Use of overall mean attitude scores calculated from the SAQ data was the main sampling technique used.

The mean institutional SAQ scores are given in figure 5.1. High, high/medium, medium, low/medium and low scores are identified. These are categorized as follows:

under 13	High student-centred attitudes
14-18	Medium/high student-centred attitudes
19-23	Medium student-centred attitudes
24-28	Medium/low student-centred attitudes
over 29	Low student-centred attitudes

Note was also taken of institutions which expressed a willingness to participate further in the study. (Overall 81% of the survey sample agreed to participate further in the study.)

Institutions selected to participate in the pilot study were chosen on the basis of those that fell into high/medium, medium or low/medium categories and whether institutions had expressed a willingness to participate further in the study. Also incorporated were an inter-mix of those offering diploma and undergraduate courses. The ratio of degree and diploma courses corresponds to the national picture of an approximate ratio of 1:3 (one degree-level course to three diploma-level courses).

Interview participants were selected by institutions themselves. Initial contact was made by telephone to senior education managers. A brief outline of aims of the study were given and managers asked if it was possible to nominate a nurse teacher interviewee. A researcher preference was identified that ideally interviewees should be someone in regular teaching contact with pre-registration nursing students and willing on a voluntary basis to be interviewed by the researcher. Assurances regarding ethical dimensions of the study were given. For example, confidentiality for institutions and interviewees was guaranteed. All institutions approached said they were able to nominate a nurse teacher/teacher interviewee.

	Attitude Scores																												
	11	12	13	14	15	16	17	18	19	20	21	22	23	24	25	26	27	28	29	30	31	32	33	34	35	36	37	38	39
I	**62#**	57	**32#**	**72**	50	**9#**	55	**78***	**28**	**80**	35	84	**48**	**54**	**37**	**51**	**89***		**7#**					**70#**					**34#**
n	**59#**	27		**63**	**68**	**44**	**78**	**86#**	**25**	**3**	**42**	**83**	**15**	17	71	**85#**		**29#**	**81#**										
s	**4**			**29#**	86#	**40**	**21***		**53**	**12**	58	**22#**	**31**	26	**67**	**3**													
t				**49**	75				**74**	10	**87**	76	**6**	**39**	**65**														
i									**43**	**69**		**61**	**5**		**90***														
t									14	**60**		**64**	**8**																
u										**24#**		**46**																	
t										**23**		**45**																	
i												**33**																	
o												16																	
n												**2#**																	
s												**88***																	
	High Student Centredness			Medium/High Student-Centredness					Medium Student-Centredness					Medium/Low Student-Centredness					Low Student-Centredness										

Interview sample

Pilot study *
Main study #

Bold print indicates those willing to participate further in the study

Figure 5.1 Institutions' mean SAQ scores and selection of the nurse teacher sample

Interviewees were contacted personally by the researcher regarding setting a date, time and place for the interview, which was confirmed by letter. Also included in confirmation letters was written information about the study and further assurances regarding maintaining confidentiality for both the interviewee and institution.

Five pilot nurse teacher interviews were conducted which were each scheduled to last one hour. The actual interviews, however, varied in length from 20 minutes to over an hour. A focused tape-recorded interview technique was used, as described by Polit and Hungler (1991). The primary task of the researcher was seen as putting interviewees at ease so they would feel comfortable in expressing honest answers. It was considered important that the researcher would appear unbiased. This was achieved by asking open questions on topic areas and receiving answers in a neutral fashion.

Analysis of the pilot study nurse teacher interview data

Tape recordings of the interviews were transcribed verbatim by the researcher. Line, page numbers, institutional and interview codes were incorporated for later cross-referencing purposes. Content analysis of the transcriptions was undertaken. Data analysis was done using a word processor which had a block, cut and paste facility. The method used is described by Burnard (1994). Each transcription was examined and meaning units identified. A meaning units is defined as a discrete phase, sentence or series of sentences which covered one idea or one related set of perceptions. These meaning units were then assigned to an appropriate category and the categories to an appropriate theme.

Levels of the content analysis of the nurse teacher data are therefore as follows:

Theme	- Major focuses of the analysis
Category	- A sub-section of a theme
Meaning Unit	- A phrase, sentence or series of sentences which gives a perceived attribute of the category

It should, however, be noted that whilst analysis is presented in a linear format the reality of analysis was that it occurred in a cyclical fashion. For example, it was possible to identify some themes and categories at the outset of analysis. However, other themes and categories emerged not as the result of direct interview questions and were only identified when meaning units were highlighted. Therefore establishing themes, categories and meaning units was done through alternating back and forth between reading the transcriptions, highlighting the meaning units and establishing themes and categories. Figure 5.2 gives the themes and data categories established from the nurse teacher interview data.

It can be demonstrated that most of the major themes reflect the structure of the interview schedule. However the theme of the role of the nurse teacher can be seen to be an implicit rather than explicit focus of the interview schedule. Also some data categories do not stem from direct interview questions. For example, clinical credibility of nurse teachers and clinical link systems were not subjects of direct interview questions in the pilot study. However, it can be seen that the majority of the interview data was obtained through an analytical deductive approach. For example, the framework of tne interview schedule was pre-determined by the researcher and based on theories of student-centred learning and teaching and patient-centred care as developed out of the literature review. A deductive approach is in keeping with the research framework of this study. For example, analysis of data is not principally aimed at generating theory but at illuminating relationships. This is compatible with the methodological triangulation research design being utilised in this study. For example, subsequent comparisons to be made between all the data sets are designed to be essentially descriptive and illuminative.

Analysis of the pilot study interview data at a meaning unit level also gave major insights into the central research question, this being whether nurse teachers act as role models for student nurses when learning about approaches to care delivery and the part student-centred learning and teaching plays in this conundrum. For example, it was said by a number of interviewees that whether nurse teachers are seen as role models for students nurses is dependent on nurse teachers' clinical credibility and if teachers undertake clinical teaching with students. Caring behaviour exhibited by teachers to students, in contrast to specific teaching and learning methods, was cited by one interviewee as being important. Therefore through analysis of the meaning units further categories emerged relating to nurse teachers as 'carers of students', their clinical roles and clinical link systems.

From the results of this data analysis the original interview schedule was modified. Certain topics were omitted. For example, questions pertaining to qualities of a good nurse were omitted as the question was felt to be too cliched and of little relevance to the study. Correspondingly certain areas were introduced. For example, roles of nurse teachers in clinical areas and clinical link systems were included. Also questions regarding manifestations of teacher caring behaviour to students were introduced.

The framework of the interviews was also modified through reflection on how the pilot study interviews had been conducted. The final interview schedule was designed to have a number of lead questions. Lead questions were open questions in response to which interviewees would be encouraged to talk as freely as possible. Dependent on responses a number of probes or clarifying questions would be posed. Probe questions relate to giving examples or justification for interviewees' responses.

The main study nurse teacher interview schedule is given in appendix 3.

Analysis of the main study nurse teacher interview data

The nurse teacher main study interview sample was selected in a similar fashion to that of the pilot study sample. Fifteen institutions were selected on the basis of their mean SAQ scores, the type of nurse education courses offered (pre-diploma, diploma or undergraduate) and their willingness to participate. All institutions approached put forward volunteers who were willing to take part in the study.

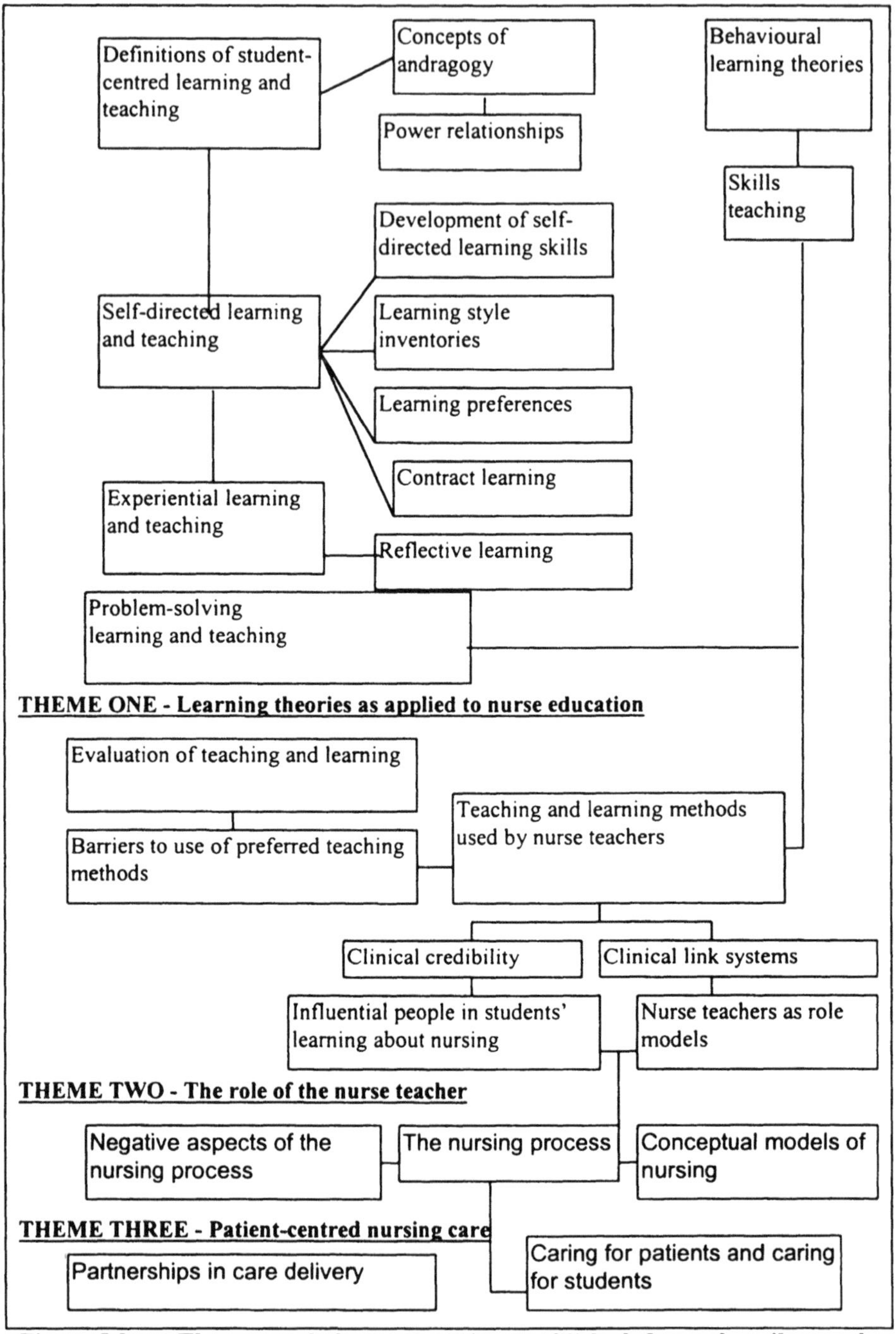

Figure 5.2 Themes and data categories established from the pilot study nurse teacher data

Details of the nurse teacher interview sample are given in appendix 4 and discussed in detail in the following chapter.

As with the pilot study all the main study interviews were tape recorded and transcribed verbatim by the researcher. Line, page numbers, institutional and interviewee codes were incorporated for cross referencing purposes.

Development of data themes and categories

Analysis of the main study interview data was conducted in a similar fashion to the pilot study data analysis. It was found that, whilst major themes remained the same, further data categories could be identified. The majority of the new categories emerged from direct questions. For example, in the pilot study it was seen that how student nurses learn about nursing was a key area and related to the caring features of the nurse teacher's role. Therefore caring for students operationalised through personal tutor systems emerged as a new data category. Establishing student group characteristics and whether these are more important to teachers than individual student characteristics is a further example. Some categories did not, however, emerge in response to direct questions. For instance monitoring attendance was identified as being inter–related to nurse teacher/student nurse power relationships.

A further stage of data of analysis was undertaken once the meaning units had been ascribed to the various categories. This final stage of analysis involved the researcher attributing descriptive phrases to each group or individual meaning units. (Where similar responses occurred meaning units are grouped together within the categories.) Both the pilot study and main study data were included in this analysis. The rationale for including both sets of data was that the data categories established in the pilot study were essentially the same as the main study categories. Furthermore the data was derived from similar interview questions. Therefore exclusion of valuable and interesting data from the main study analysis was thought to be unjustified.

Data tables were then compiled with numerical values given to each ascribed feature (meaning unit interpretation) of a category. Presenting the data in such a fashion is designed to synthesise them into a manageable and more easily comprehended format.

Results of this analysis of the nurse teacher interview data are presented in the following chapter.

Student nurse questionnaire

The final phase of the data collection is of conducting a survey of pre–registration student nurses' attitudes towards student–centred learning and teaching and patient–centred nursing care. Aims of this part of the data collection therefore address the final two research questions. There is an implicit aim of this section of data collection to continue to collect data of both a qualitative and quantitative nature. However, resourcing issues made separate visits to collect two sets of data impossible. It was not, for example possible to continue to take a national survey approach and make separate visits in order to conduct both in–depth student nurse interviews and also to administer the PMQX instrument. Difficulties gaining access to pre–registration student were also envisaged. For example, it was thought that permission to conduct the research might be required from some institutions' educational ethical committees. Also it was thought that classroom time–tabling might make scheduling of visits to administer the questionnaire and also conduct in–depth interviews difficult. It therefore was decided to incorporate the PMQX instrument into an open–ended questionnaire regarding student–centred learning and teaching. It was thought that by adopting this approach data collection would be a relatively simple exercise but still yield a fairly good amount of both qualitative and quantitative data. However, as discussed later in this chapter the instrument eventually used for this part of the study was quite lengthy. It was also estimated that it could take a relatively long time to complete, which possibly could affect completion rates.

Development of the student nurse questionnaire

As stated previously the student nurse questionnaire had two discrete parts. The first part was that of incorporating statements relating to student–centred learning and teaching to which respondents were to be invited to make comments upon. These statements mirrored the statements and questions in the SAQ survey and the nurse teacher interviews. Therefore it is believed that further methodological and data triangulation is incorporated in the study. For example, when conducting data analysis it was thought it would be possible to compare data obtained from the differing perspectives of nurse teachers and pre–registration student nurses. These data sets could also be compared to the SAQ data.

Design of the statements in the first part of the student nurse questionnaire was directed towards keeping them simple and clear. The first 6 statements addressed the main areas of student–centred learning as identified from the review of the literature. Statements were included which related to self–directed, experiential and problem–solving learning and teaching, student learning and teaching preferences and concepts of andragogy. The statements related to whether it was believed by respondents that these areas of learning and teaching are incorporated into their courses, what were respondents' preferred learning and teaching methods, and whether it was felt by respondents that were treated as adults by the majority of people they had come into contact whilst on their course. Responses to these statements, it was believed, could be compared to both the attitude survey and interview data.

Further statements were designed to examine what the student nurses believed is the most effective way of learning about nursing. Responses to these statements, it was thought, would reveal how important classroom teaching regarding nursing was in comparison with learning in clinical areas. Therefore again responses could be compared to the nurse teacher interview data, especially in terms of the nurse teacher's role in clinical teaching.

Final statements related to who were seen as being the most influential when learning about nursing, and whether students felt they were valued by people they had come into contact with whilst on their course. The first of these statements addresses role imitation theory as discussed in earlier parts of this study. It was thought that responses to these statements would give insight into who the most powerful role models are for students in the sample when they are learning about nursing. The final statement related to being valued as an individual and would give insight into the value (or non–value) of meaningful interpersonal relationships when student nurses are learning to care for patients. Also it would give some indication of the students' self–esteem. For example, positive responses regarding being valued as an individual would give some indication of positive self–esteem.

The second part of the questionnaire centred on use of the Patient–Centredness Multi–Choice Questionnaire (PMQX). The PMQX was identified during the literature search as one that would possibly address potential research questions regarding patient–centred care. The author of the questionnaire was contacted and a request made for a copy of the instrument. The PMQX and its reported validity and reliability of the instrument were subsequently examined.

The design of the PMQX instrument is described by Rolfe (1993b). The PMQX is intended measure Rogers' attitudes of empathy, genuineness and respect. The test gives patient care vignettes to which there are various reply options. The test is relatively short, with 10 items included, and reports to measure an overall therapeutic attitude of patient–centredness.

Rolfe (1993b) states that both validity and reliability issues have been addressed in development the test. For example, the PMQ was validated against a test already shown to have been both valid and reliable, namely the BLRI (Barrett–Lennard Relationship Inventory). The BLRI (Barrett–Lennard 1962), although both valid and reliable and correlating significantly with therapeutic outcomes, was considered too long for practical use and not directly applicable to the experiences of nurses. Rolfe reports that an 18 item version of the PMQ and BLRI were administered to a sample group of 94 nursing students in the first year of Project 2000 training. It was found that there was a highly significant correlation between the global attitude of patient–centredness as measured by the PMQ and general attitudes represented by the average score on the BLRI.

The reliability of the PMQ test was estimated through computation of the test–retest coefficient. The validated PMQX was administered to a group of 87 Project 2000 students who had completed 4 months of their course. The same test was readministered 3 weeks later and results compared. A test–retest reliability coefficient of 0.86 was obtained. This value was considered by its author to be adequate.

Having validated the PMQX the author piloted the instrument on a sample group of 327 student nurses. Subsequent statistical analysis of the PMQX scores showed the scores obtained to follow generally a normal distribution curve. The scores were reported to range from a minimum of 25, which is below the author's estimates of a minimally therapeutic range, to a maximum of 47 which is considered significantly therapeutic. It was concluded by the author that the PMQX discriminates between respondents in a statistically acceptable manner.

Having investigated the reported validity and reliability of the PMQX it was judged as being appropriate for use in this study. The author was then contacted again in order to gain permission to use the instrument in this study. Permission was subsequently given.

The student–centred learning statements and the PMQX were then incorporated into a questionnaire to which were added questions relating to respondents' biographical details. These details included sex, age, year of study, branch option and academic level of the course. It was planned to use these details as independent variables in subsequent statistical analysis.

Final consideration of the pilot study questionnaire was undertaken in order to make it visually interesting and thereby increase respondent motivation to complete it. To this end some illustrations were included on the front cover of the questionnaire.

Pilots study of the student nurse questionnaire

The aim of the pilot study was to test the appropriateness of the general presentation of the questionnaire. There was also an intention to identify difficulties with completion of the first part of the questionnaire with regard to perceptions of student–centred learning and teaching. The final aim was to obtain an estimate of the time required by the student nurses to complete the questionnaire. As the PMQX had already been subjected to reliability and validity testing by its author, further pre–tests were considered unnecessary.

The nurse education institutions which had participated in the nurse teacher interviews were to be used to obtain samples for the pilot and main study of the student nurse questionnaire. It was thought that this would enable relatively easy access to student groups. For example, it is shown later in the study that all the nurse teachers interviewed thought it would be possible for the researcher to gain access to a small group of student nurses in their educational establishment. It was thought, however, by some of the interviewees that permission would be needed from their educational ethical committee in addition to the College Principal or equivalent. However all the interviewees offered help in facilitating access.

The institutions approached regarding participation in the pilot study were selected on the criteria that they had obtained medium and medium high scores on of their institution's SAQ. A general overview of selection of both the pilot and main study student nurse questionnaire samples is given in Figure 5.3.

The rationale for inclusion of medium and a medium high scoring institutions was, that it was envisaged that it possibly would be difficult to access high and low range scoring institutions' student nurse groups, because, as with any normal distribution curve, there are relatively few institutions at each extreme of the curve.

It was, however, seen as important to incorporate a major difference in terms of academic level of the course into the pilot study. Therefore one group of student nurses participating in the pilot study was undertaking an undergraduate degree programme and the other a diploma programme. This was considered important as it was hoped the pilot study would reveal any non–understanding or misunderstanding of the terms used in the first part of the questionnaire. So, for example, although sophisticated terms such as experiential learning were not being used, it was hoped that any lack of general understanding of other more simple terms would be revealed.

It was thought that differing standards of the students' educational programme could possibly be a factor in this understanding or non–understanding.

Initial contact with the institutions selected for the pilot study was made through the nurse teacher interviewees. A letter was sent to the person the interviewee thought was most appropriate in order to obtain permission for the study. Both institutions approached agreed to participate in the pilot study. Neither required ethical committee permission for access to a student sample.

The samples for the pilot study of the student nurse questionnaire were selected by the educational establishment themselves. They were therefore convenience samples. A request was made for access to a small group of Common Foundation Programme students (around 10 students in total). There were 2 pilot sample groups of pre–registration student nurses (n=13 and n=18). One group was in their third year of training and the other in their second. All the student nurses in the sample were undertaking adult nurse training. These sample were larger than those identified as the ideal and one group was further on in their training than the requested group of Common Foundation Programme students. However, neither of these factors were seen as making substantial differences to achieving the aims of the pilot study.

Pilot study of the student nurse questionnaire – data collection

Having gained permission to conduct the pilot study in the two institutions, arrangements for access to the students were made. At the data collection visits initial explanations regarding the purpose of the study were given to the two student groups. Whilst it had been requested that the students be told prior to the data collection visit that their participation in the study was entirely voluntary this was repeated. Also the usual reassurances were given in terms of the researcher maintaining both the anonymity of respondents and their institution and that all responses obtained would remain confidential to the researcher.

All the student nurses in the diploma group agreed to take part in the study. The total size of this group was 20. Two students were absent from the class and so the overall response rate was therefore 90% (n=18). However, under half of the undergraduates student nurses agreed to participate. The total size of this group was 27, and the overall response rate was 48.15% (n=13). Reasons for the lack of enthusiasm to participate by the undergraduates was thought to relate to the fact that the questionnaire was being distributed in one of the last sessions of the academic year.

The student nurses were requested when completing the questionnaire to ask for clarification if anything was unclear. Grammatical and typographical errors were subsequently pointed out by both the student groups. Also a number of questions were asked by the students which related, for example, to what was meant by some of the statements. It was felt, however, that it was not non–understanding or misunderstanding of the statements that was at issue. Generally it appeared that the students in the pilot study groups saw the questionnaire as a test of knowledge, with only 'right' answers being sought by the researcher as against personal beliefs and values of respondents. This did not appear to invalidate any of the statements or their wording but did indicate that in the main study careful instructions needed to be given that it was personal beliefs and opinions that were being sought.

Minimum and maximum times for completion of the questionnaire were also noted. These were 20 minutes to 1 hour. The early finishers were found to be a problem in the diploma student group as they appeared reluctant to leave without been given permission. Therefore it was noted for the main study respondents would need to be told beforehand that they could leave but to do so as quietly as possible so as not to disturb the remainder of the group.

Data analysis of the student nurse questionnaire

Data analysis of the pilot data was initially directed towards examining responses obtained to the statements pertaining to student–centred learning. The general approach taken was that of a content analysis. For example, responses to each of the statements given in the questionnaire were initially transcribed verbatim. These were subsequently analysed in order to establish major groupings of responses to each question.

The final stage of analysis of the student–centred learning data obtained in the pilot study was to make some preliminary comparisons with that of the SAQ survey data and nurse teacher interview data. It was found that it was possible to undertake a comparative analysis, and meaningful triangulation of all the sets of data obained would therefore be achieved. However, it was identified that there was a major omission in terms of the questions given on the student nurse questionnaire as compared to the other sets of data. This omission related to how student nurses define student–centred learning. Therefore a further statement was added to the first part of the questionnaire.

The second stage of data analysis was directed towards examining the responses to the PMQX. As said earlier, it was not considered necessary to undertaken any statistical analysis of the PMQX regarding the instrument's validity and reliability as this had shown to be satisfactory by its author. The pilot study analysis was therefore directed towards formulating data coding categories and examination of response rates.

Examination of response rates to the PMQX showed them to be consistently lower than those of the first section of the questionnaire. For example, one institution had a response rate of 37.00% as compared to 48.15% for the first part of the questionnaire. The other sample group had a 85.00% PMQX response rate which could be compared to a response rate of 90.00% for the second part of the questionnaire. It was felt that these differences in response rates were due to the concerns raised earlier regarding the overall length of the questionnaire. These concerns had been compounded by, as discussed previously, the addition of a further question to the first part of the questionnaire. Examination of individual questionnaires revealed generally that those who had completed the PMQX section tended not to have answered the student–centred learning section in quite so much detail.

Appendix 5 gives the final version of the student nurse questionnaire.

Student nurse questionnaire survey – main study

An initial issue when considering the main study student nurse questionnaire survey was selection of the research sample. It was discovered in the pilot study that the potential amount of data that could be obtained from a single data collection visit was relatively large. It was therefore decided to select a further sub–sample from institutions who had participated in the nurse teacher interviews. It was thought originally that an ideal number would be 10 institutions with 10 respondents completing the questionnaire from each institution. It was envisaged that data from this sample would give reasonable and manageable amounts of qualitative and quantitative data. For example, a sample of 100 would enable meaningful statistical analysis of the PMQX data and at the same time the qualitative data from the student–centred section would be reasonably manageable.

A questionnaire survey of 100 student nurse respondents who were towards the end of their Common Foundation Programme was therefore the intention. The decision to include only Common Foundation Programme students was made on the basis of a desire to compare data from students at a similar stage of training and so that a meaningful comparison could be made to SAQ survey scores.

Selection of the institutions to be approached for the student nurse survey was similar to that of the nurse teacher sample. Institutions were selected on the criteria of their SAQ scores and academic levels of their pre–registration programmes. Institutions were therefore approached that had high, medium high, medium, medium low and low SAQ scores. An inter–mix of institutions offering diploma and degree level were also approached. The inter–mix was to take account of the differing numbers of degree and diploma courses offered nationally, an approximate ratio being 1 degree level course to 3 diploma level courses. From experiences accrued from the nurse teacher interviews it was thought unlikely that it would be possible to gain access to a student group undertaking pre–Project 2000 training due to the rarity of these courses. Therefore it was decided not to include students undergoing this type of training. All the educational institutions approached agreed to provide access to a student group. None required ethical committee permission to conduct the study.

Figure 5.3 gives an overview of the selection of pilot and main study student nurse survey samples.

Analysis of the main study student nurse questionnaire data

It was found that a number of the educational institutions approached arranged access to student groups who were far in excess of the number of students requested. For example the largest student group from any one institution was in excess of 50 students. The eventual sample was 224 out of a total population of 302 and the response rate was therefore 74.17%. However, this response rate refers to the percentage of respondents from the total population and is therefore deceptive. For example, in majority of instances students were absent from the day's teaching sessions and therefore were considered to be part of the total student group population but were not present to complete the questionnaire. Apart from a group of student nurses in the pilot study, no students present at data collection sessions refused to participate. However, as with the pilot study it was stressed that their participation was entirely voluntary. Also assurances of anonymity and confidentiality were also given.

Whilst the eventual sample of 224 was far in excess of the originally intended sample size this was, however, not seen as affecting the results of the study. For example, the main intention of having a relatively small sample size was in order to limit the amount of qualitative data obtained, and therefore keep data analysis manageable. It is thought that the larger than planned sample size gives greater reliability to both the qualitative and quantitative data analysis. For example, Polit and Hungler (1991) relate that researchers should use the largest sample possible, as the larger the sample, the more representative of the population it is likely to be.

The amount of data obtained from of the student centred learning and teaching section of the questionnaire, therefore, was potentially difficult manage in respect of the qualitative data obtained from the first section of the questionnaire. Handling of the data was, however, to some extent simplified by taking a content analysis approach. For example, although individual unique responses were incorporated where possible into data analysis the main intention of analysis was to look for majority shared beliefs, this being in keeping with taking a survey approach in examining beliefs and attitudes to student–centred learning in pre–registration nurse education.

As with the pilot study, all the responses to the first part of the student nurse questionnaire were transcribed verbatim. Subsequently a content analysis of the data was undertaken. Similar responses were grouped together. Researcher descriptions were given and ascribed to each data group. This analysis was done initially on an institution to institution basis so as to enable comparisons between the responses of the various student nurse groups. However, all the data obtained was eventually merged together into a table format, each set of data corresponding to a question posed on the first section of the student nurse questionnaire.

The results of the analysis of the student-centred learning and teaching section of the student nurse survey questionnaire is given in the following chapter.

Attitude Scores	11	12	13	14	15	16	17	18	19	20	21	22	23	24	25	26	27	28	29	30	31	32	33	34	35	36	37	38	39
I	**62**	**57**	**32#**	**72**	50	**79#**	55	**78***	**28**	**80**	35	84	**48**	**54**	**37**	**51**	**89#**		**7#**			**70**						**34***	
n	**59#**	27		**63**	**68**	**44**	**78**	**86**	**25**	73	**42**	**83**	**15**	**17**	71	**85**	**29**		**81**										
s	**4**			**29**	18	**40**		**21#**	**53**	**12**	58	**22**	**31**	26	**67**	**3**													
t				**49**	75				**74**	10	**87**	76	**6**	**39**	**65**														
i									**43**	**69**	**61**	**5**			**90#**														
t									**14**	**60**	**64**	**8**																	
u										**24***	**46**																		
t										**23**	**45**																		
i											**33**																		
o											16																		
n											**2#**																		
s											**88#**																		
	High Student-Centredness			Medium/High Student-Centredness					Medium Student-Centredness					Medium/Low Student-Centredness					Low Student-Centredness										

Interview sample
Pilot study *
Main study #
Bold print indicates those willing to participate further in the study

Figure 5.3 Institutions' mean SAQ scores and selection of the student nurse sample

PMQX data analysis

The second part of the student nurse survey questionnaire relates to PMQX estimates. In the PMQX section of the questionnaire the response rate was 192 (63.58%). This response rate is approximately 10% less than for the first section of the questionnaire. Incompletely answered or spoilt responses account for this lower response rate.

Specific difficulties were encountered regarding the data collection for this section of the student nurse questionnaire For example, whilst only student groups who were in the middle or towards the end of their Common Foundation Programme studies were requested, often it was necessary to conduct the research with student groups who did not fit with the pre–determined criteria. Reasons for this stemmed mainly from being allocated access time to student groups in often very full timetables. Also student groups were sometimes inaccessible as a whole group when undertaking clinical placements. Therefore it was necessary to broaden the sample criteria to include student groups at different points of their pre–registration courses. Students at the beginning of their studies, at the end of their studies and students from different branches eventually formed part of the sample. Whilst initially this was seen as potentially presenting difficulties in terms of comparing 'like with like' subsequent data analysis revealed that it was possible to compare responses to the PMQX section of the questions using a greater variety of independent variables than originally envisaged.

Generally the PMQX main study data were analysed in a similar fashion to the pilot study data. The data were data coded both with regards to the biographical details of the respondents, academic levels of the pre–registration programmes being undertaking, branch studies and stage of training of respondents. Individual and institutional global scores of patient–centredness were also computed.

Appendix 6 gives the respondent details to the student nurse questionnaire.

The PMQX data were subsequently analysed using SPSSX. The results of this analysis are presented in the following chapter of this study.

6 Results of the study

The subject matter of this chapter is analysis of the research data. Data analysis initially focuses on results of the SAQ survey. Later sections of the chapter examine data obtained from the nurse teacher interviews and student nurse questionnaires.

SAQ survey data analysis

As described in the previous chapter the initial part of this study centred on a survey of attitudes regarding student–centred learning using the SAQ instrument. The sample was drawn from the total population of educational institutions undertaking pre–registration nurse education in England. Items on the SAQ were developed from key themes identified in a review of the published literature on the topic area. Also described in previous chapters were how data coding was undertaken and how the SAQ data were subsequently analysed using SPSSX.

Statistical methods used in the first part of analysis of the SAQ survey data fall within the general remit of descriptive statistics. Later sections of the analysis will, however, have as their focus the use of inferential statistics.

Central to the use of descriptive statistics are estimations of frequency distributions, measures of central tendency and variability. Frequency distributions allow structure to be imposed on data. Measures of central tendency are considered through analysis of mean and median scores. The purpose of this analysis is to estimate the average or central values. It is, however, recognised that whilst measures of central tendency are important, averages do not give the total picture of distribution. Therefore variability between the scores are demonstrated through analysis of standard deviation scores.

Statistical analysis of the SAQ survey – frequencies, means, medians and standard deviations

Results of data analysis of the SAQ survey pertaining to frequency distribution, means, medians and standard deviations is given in table 6.1.

Attitude 1 pertains to whether the principles of teaching adults differ from those of teaching children. Table 6.1 shows generally that there are high agreement scores with to this attitude statement. For example, 65 respondents (85.525%) agree or strongly agree that principles of teaching adults differ from teaching children. This also may be demonstrated by high agreement of mean and median scores. However, 8 respondents (10.525%) disagree or strongly disagree with the statement. The variation in responses is demonstrated by a moderately high standard deviation. Overall there is a pattern of high agreement scores with the statement.

Data analysis with respect to attitude 2 also shows a high agreement score, with 72 (94.078%) of respondents agreeing that self–directed learning is an important feature of student–centred learning and teaching. A small number of respondents (5.262%) disagreed with the statement. However, there is only a small amount of variance in responses which is demonstrated by the relatively low standard deviation. Finally, that there are no mid–range scores may be seen to demonstrate a lack of ambivalence in the way respondents scored their responses to this attitude statement.

Responses to attitude 3 again shows high agreement scores. For example 67 respondents (88.157%) agreed that self–directed learning skills are taught in the institution's pre–registration nurse education programme compared to a small proportion who disagreed with the statement (5.262%). A relatively low standard deviation score demonstrates little variability in the overall pattern of scores. As with a number of attitudes analysed, there are relatively small numbers of mid–range scores which demonstrates little ambivalence in the ways respondents have scored their responses.

In contrast to the attitude scores analysed previously response to attitude statement 4 demonstrates relatively less agreement with the statement that regular account is taken of students' learning styles in the institution's pre–registration teaching sessions. Also shown is the fact that, although there are 39 (51.314%) in agreement with the statement there are fewer respondents strongly agreeing as against merely agreeing. However, mean and median scores, whilst lower than those of those given previously, still demonstrate general agreement with the statement. It is evident also that there is a grouping of middle scores, for example, there is a mid range score of 21 (27.631%). These neutral responses may indicate either poor statement construction or non–understanding of what is meant by learning styles. In contrast there are 16 (21.052%) respondents who are in disagreement with the statement. However, none strongly disagree. This moderately high variation of scores is demonstrated by a standard deviance of 1.039.

Responses to attitude 5 demonstrates a similar overall picture to that of attitude 4, the major difference being that of slightly higher agreement scores – 43 (56.578%) responses. However, these responses are represented by more agreement than strong agreement values. There are moderately high proportions of mid–range responses (21.052%) and disagreement responses (22.368%). Similarity of responses between attitudes 4 and 5 may be reflected in similarities of subject areas of each statement. It may therefore be concluded that there is evidence that there is a blurring of how learning styles and learning preferences are defined.

Table 6.1
Frequencies, percentage frequencies, mean, median and standard deviation of responses to the attitude statements

Attitude statements	Value	Frequ	%	Mean	Median	SD
1. The principles of teaching adults differ from teaching children	1	43	56.578%	1.724	1	1.078
	2	22	28.947%			
	3	3	3.947%			
	4	5	6.578%			
	5	3	3.947%			
2. Self-directed learning is an important feature of student-centred learning and teaching	1	47	61.184%	1.513	1	0.806
	2	25	32.894%			
	3	0	0.000%			
	4	2	2.631%			
	5	2	2.631%			
3. Self-directed study skills are taught in the institution's pre-registration nurse education programme	1	41	53.947%	1.658	1	0.917
	2	26	34.210%			
	3	5	6.578%			
	4	2	2.631%			
	5	2	2.631%			
4. Regular account is taken of students' learning styles in teaching sessions in the institution's pre-registration nurse education programme	1	15	19.736%	2.50	2	1.039
	2	24	31.578%			
	3	21	27.631%			
	4	16	21.052%			
	5	0	0.000%			

Table 6.1 cont:

Attitude statements	Value	Frequ	%	Mean	Median	SD
5. Regular account is taken of students' learning preferences in teaching sessions in the institution's pre-registration nurse education programme	1 2 3 4 5	11 32 16 17 0	14.473% 42.105% 21.052% 22.368% 0.000%	2.513	2	1.000
6. Contract learning is used regularly in the institution's pre-registration nurse education programme	1 2 3 4 5	20 24 5 20 7	26.315% 31.578% 6.578% 26.315% 9.210%	2.605	2	1.367
7. Student-centred learning means active learning	1 2 3 4 5	44 20 5 4 3	57.894% 26.315% 6.578% 5.263% 3.947%	1.711	1	1.069
8. Nurse teachers negotiate with students in regard of the teaching and learning methods they use in the institutions's pre-registration nurse education programme	1 2 3 4 5		31.578% 39.473% 14.473% 13.157% 1.315%	2.131	2	1.050

Table 6.1 cont:

Attitude statements	Value	Frequ	%	Mean	Median	SD
9. Student nurses are encouraged to reflect on their clinical experiences undertaken in the institution's pre-registration education programme	1 2 3 4 5	50 23 1 0 2	65.789% 30.263% 1.315% 0.000% 2.631%	1.434	1	0.772
10. Student-centred learning and teaching involves problem-solving activities	1 2 3 4 5	56 20 0 0 0	73.684% 26.315% 0.000% 0.000% 0.000%	1.263	1	0.443
11. Critical thinking skills are a valued educational outcome of the institution's pre-registration nurse education programme	 1 2 3 4 5	53 20 0 1 2	69.736% 26.315% 0.000% 1.315% 2.631%	1.408	1	0.803

Table 6.1 gives 44 (57.89%) respondents agreeing with the statement that contract learning is used regularly in the institution's pre–registration nurse education programme. However, a larger proportion of scores are of agreement (24 responses – 31.578%) as against those of strong agreement (20 responses – 26.315%). General agreement with the statement is also demonstrated by the mean score of 2.605. However, this statement has the highest mean score obtained for any of the attitude scores and therefore is the statement which has the least agreement scores. There are few mid–range scores (5 responses – 6.578%) but relatively high disagreement scores (27 responses – 35.525%). Finally the responses give rise to the highest standard deviation score which demonstrates a degree of greater variation. However, this variation contrasts in agreement or disagreement to the statement rather than mid–range, neutral responses.

Responses to attitude 7 demonstrates high agreement scores, with 64 (84.209%) of the respondents agreeing that student–centred learning means active learning. General agreement is also shown in the relatively low mean agreement score of 1.069. This may be compared to 7 responses (9.210%) who disagree with the statement. However, there is a moderately high standard deviation of 1.069. There is, for example, a greater variation in responses than to other statements. There are also 5 responses (6.578%) who give mid–range neutral responses.

There are also high agreement scores (54 responses – 71.051%) with the attitude statement that nurse teachers negotiate with pre–registration student nurses with regard to teaching and learning methods they use. This agreement score is, however, characterized by proportionally more agreement scores (30 responses – 39.473%) than strongly agree scores (24 responses – 31.473%). There are also relatively more mid–range responses (11 responses – 14.473%) than to some other attitudes statements which indicates more unsure, neutral responses. Whilst 11 respondents disagree with the statement there is only 1 respondent (1.315%) in the strong disagreement category. Lack of strong disagreement responses is, however, a feature of responses to all the attitude statements.

Responses to attitude statement 9 demonstrates the highest agreement score so far, with 73 (96.052%) agreeing that student nurses are encouraged to reflect on their clinical experiences. Moreover the majority of these agreement scores fall into the strong agreement category (50 responses – 65.789%). There are very few mid–range responses (1 response – 1.315%) and disagreement responses (2 responses – 2.631%).

The data given in table 6.1 with respect to attitude 10 shows the highest and most unequivocal agreement response with any of the attitude statements. All the respondents agreed or strongly agreed with the statement that student–centred learning means problem–solving learning. The majority of responses are of strong agreement category (56 responses –73.684%).

As with previous responses to the attitude statements, the responses to attitude 11 demonstrates high agreement scores (73 responses – 96.051%) with the statement that critical thinking skills are a valued educational outcome of the institution's pre–registration nurse education programme. There are no mid–range scores and relatively few disagreement scores (3 responses – 3.946%).

Summary of the descriptive statistics section regarding the SAQ data

Generally the initial stage of analysis of the SAQ survey data gives a picture of overall agreement with the attitude statements. Strong agreement with statements is demonstrated related to concepts identified in the literature review about how student–centred learning is defined with regard to nurse education. For example, there are general agreement scores with the statements that the principles of teaching children differs from those of teaching adults, and self–directed learning, active learning and problem–solving learning are part of student–centred learning. High agreement scores were obtained with regard to self–directed study skills being taught in pre–registration nurse education programmes the institutions surveyed. Also shown is general agreement with the value of reflection on clinical practice and critical thinking skills as an important educational outcome of pre–registration nurse education programmes. Mid–range scores were obtained with regard to regular account being taken of students' learning styles and learning preferences and that contract learning is used regularly in the institutions surveyed.

It may therefore be concluded from these results that the SAQ respondents value concepts of treating student nurses as adults and principles of student–centred learning and teaching. However, there is less evidence that the humanistic philosophies underpinning these concepts and principles are actually articulated in nurse education programmes. For example, there is less value placed by respondents on negotiation with regard to teaching and learning methods and taking account of individual differences in learning styles and preferences. However, there is evidence that the skills needed for self–directed learning are seen as being developed in nurse education programmes. Certain educational outcomes seen as important for post–registration nursing practice may also be identified as being valued by the respondents. These include critical and reflective thinking skills.

SAQ survey sample details

The following analysis of the attitude survey data relates to responses made to the attitude statements and their relationship to the characteristics of the SAQ survey respondents. The biographical and institutional details are given in appendix 2.

Generally respondents to the SAQ survey comprised largely of females (52 respondents – 68.421%), those aged between 40–49 years (48 respondents – 63.157%) and those who had been qualified as a nurse teacher for over ten years (53 respondents – 69.736%). The most under–represented in the sample are therefore males (24 respondent – 31.578%), those aged between 20–29 years (0 respondents) and those who might be described as unqualified nurse teachers (1 respondent – 1.315%). The positions respondents held within the various educational institutions were slightly more difficult to analyse due to the multiplicity of differing job titles used. However, the majority of the respondents gave their job title as one usually associated with senior educational management roles within nurse education institutions (45 respondents – 59.210%).

The SAQ sample profile can be seen to provide a broad fit with the aims of this stage of the research which is to obtain a general picture of attitudes to student–centred learning from senior educational managers in institutions conducting pre–registration nurse education courses in England. However, as identified, in the pilot study the largest portion of responses obtained to the attitude survey were from those in upper middle management positions in nurse education institutions rather than from those in top management positions.

Characteristics of the pre–registration nurse education courses offered by the SAQ respondents' educational institution

The academic level of courses offered by the respondents' educational institutions were in the majority diploma only courses (27 – 35.526%). This may be compared to

3 respondents (3.947%) whose institutions offered certificate level courses only and 14 responents (18.421%) whose institutions offered only undergraduate courses. However, 32 respondents (42.526%) reported that their institution offered a mix of two or more differing educational level pre–registration nurse education courses.

Cohort size was such that the majority of institutions had intake sizes of over 80 (40 respondents – 52.631%). Of these 80 respondents 17 (22.368%) reported institutional cohort sizes of over 120. In contrast 22 respondents (28.947%) estimated their institutions' cohort sizes to be under 59, with 10 respondents (13.157%) reporting cohort sizes of between 20 and 39.

Data coding of class size was, as described in the previous chapter, more difficult than with the other categories of data. The main measurement of class size was range groupings. These groupings show that 15 respondents (19.736%) give estimations of class size in their institution as being regularly 30 and under. These may be compared to 22 respondents (28.947%) who report their institution's class size may on occasions be over 100. The largest proportion of respondents, however, reported class size in their institution to be on occasion 40–79 (34.210%).

Statistical analysis of the SAQ survey

This section of the chapter focuses on statistical analysis of the SAQ survey data with regard to statistically significant responses to the SAQ statements. Differences in responses are considered in relation to a number of independent variables. The independent variables are sex, age and number of years qualified as a nurse teacher. Also considered are differences in the institutions' cohort sizes, average class sizes and educational levels of the pre–registration courses offered by the institutions.

The null hypotheses being tested are as follows:

> There are no significant differences in attitude scores in relation to the demographic variables of sex, age and number of years qualified as a nurse teacher.
>
> There are no significant differences in attitudes scores in relation to the context variables of academic level of the course, cohort size and average class size.

Data collected with regard to these independent variables can be seen to be at nominal and ordinal levels of measurement. For example, nominal (yes or no) data were collected in terms of sex and academic level of the course. Ranking or ordinal data were collected with regard to age, number of years qualified as a nurse teacher, reported class size and cohort size.

Nonparametric tests were deemed as being appropriate for use with all the data collected. It is, however, recognised that nonparametric tests require less stringent assumptions regarding the nature of the data collected and therefore are less powerful tools of analysis than parametric tests.

The level of significance was established at 0.05.

Table 6.2 gives the Mann–Whitney test results with regard to responses to the attitude statements 1–11 according to sex. Analysis of the test results show there is a significant difference pertaining to attitude 9. This difference indicates that males in the sample are shown to agree less strongly that pre–registration student nurses are encouraged to reflect on their clinical nursing experiences. There are no other significant differences.

Table 6.2
Mann–Whitney comparisons of attitudes 1–11 by sex

	U Score	2-Tailed Probability
Att 1	564.0	.4519
Att 2	613.5	.8906
Att 3	622.5	.9851
Att 4	563.5	.4834
Att 5	565.5	.4912
Att 6	525.0	.2516
Att 7	621.0	.9699
Att 8	492.5	.1218
Att 9	472.5	.0412*
Att 10	598.0	.7033
Att 11	549.0	.2958

Tables 6.3 and 6.4 give Chi–Square and Spearman's Correlation computations in regards of age. There are no significant differences in responses to attitude statement relating to age.

Table 6.3
Chi–Square comparisons of attitudes 1–11 by age

	Chi-Square	Significance
Att 1	1.3707	.5039
Att 2	1.2846	.5261
Att 3	2.9145	.1628
Att 4	.0619	.9695
Att 5	1.4395	.4869
Att 6	.0372	.9816
Att 7	1.6518	.4378
Att 8	.0458	.9749
Att 9	1.0438	.4682
Att 10	.3331	.7511
Att 11	.6986	.5807

Table 6.4
Spearman's correlation of attitudes 1–11 by age

	Coefficient
Att 1	–.0355
Att 2	–.0945
Att 3	–.0453
Att 4	0287
Att 5	–.0744
Att 6	.0151
Att 7	–.1105
Att 8	.0059
Att 9	–.1365
Att 10	–.0270
Att 11	–.1203

Table 6.5 gives data analysis results of Chi–Square comparisons with number of years qualified as a nurse teacher. There are no significant results with regard to any of the attitude statements.

Table 6.5
Chi–Square comparisons of attitudes 1–11 with number of years qualified as a nurse teacher

	Chi-Square	Significance
Att 1	1.9943	.5736
Att 2	2.3267	.5074
Att 3	3.9910	.2624
Att 4	2.7000	.4402
Att 5	3.1477	.3694
Att 6	2.0020	.5720
Att 7	1.2122	.6732
Att 8	1.8574	.5601
Att 9	1.6744	.6426
Att 10	4.1115	.2497
Att 11	.9057	.8241

Table 6.6 shows a significant difference between cohort size and attitude 4. Respondents with cohort sizes 40–59 and 60–79 are seen as being less likely to agree that regular account is taken of students' learning styles in teaching sessions in their institution's pre–registration nurse education programme. There are no further significant differences

Table 6.6
Chi–Square comparisons of attitudes 1–11 with cohort size

	Chi-Square	Significance
Att 1	9.4879	.0911
Att 2	1.0251	.9605
Att 3	5.1299	.4002
Att 4	11.0644	.0501*
Att 5	9.6443	.0860
Att 6	6.7067	.2434
Att 7	3.3982	.6388
Att 8	3.0496	.6923
Att 9	3.8454	.5719
Att 10	7.3045	.1990
Att 11	7.3045	.1990

Table 6.7 shows there are two significant results with regard to the independent variables academic levels of the pre–registration nurse education programme offered. For example, those respondents who still offer certificate level courses are more likely to disagree with the statement that principles of teaching adults differ from those of teaching children. Also respondents whose institutions conduct diploma level courses are less likely to agree with the that statement contract learning is used regularly in the institution's pre–registration nurse education course.

Table 6.7
Mann–Whitney comparisons of attitudes 1–11 with level of course

	Degree		Diploma		Certificate	
	U	2-tailed p	U	2-tailed p	U	2-tailed p
Att 1	649.5	.7857	428.5	.3073	503.0	.0412*
Att 2	569.5	.1958	480.5	.7590	646.0	.7428
Att 3	625.0	.5722	491.0	.8839	548.0	.1361
Att 4	590.0	.3600	432.5	.3726	555.0	.1915
Att 5	593.0	.3704	497.5	.9581	598.0	.4014
Att 6	671.5	.9955	349.5	.0496*	538.5	.1363
Att 7	603.0	.4024	500.0	.9832	537.0	.1014
Att 8	571.5	.2545	417.0	.2674	597.0	.3951
Att 9	625.5	.5460	478.0	.7239	636.5	.6448
Att 10	620.0	.4629	445.5	.3601	658.0	.8433
Att 11	628.0	.5545	492.0	.8826	642.0	.6870

Table 6.8 gives two significant results regarding comparisons of attitude responses with class size. For example, respondents with reported class size of on occasions 80–99 and on occasions over 100 are more likely to disagree with the statement that principles of teaching adults differ from those of teaching children. Also respondents with reported class sizes of regularly 30 and under are more likely to agree that student–centred learning means active learning.

Table 6.8
Chi–Square comparisons of attitudes 1–11 with class size

	Chi-Square	Significance
Att 1	10.1125	.0386*
Att 2	4.8937	.2984
Att 3	1.7602	.7798
Att 4	1.8732	.7591
Att 5	1.6606	.7979
Att 6	.8010	.9383
Att 7	11.0876	.0256*
Att 8	2.4664	.6507
Att 9	.9255	.9209
Att 10	.5807	.9652
Att 11	3.5081	.4766

Summary of the inferential statistical analysis of the SAQ survey data

Partial verification of the experimental hypotheses has been demonstrated in that statistically significant results have been obtained with regard to certain demographical and context variables. For example, females in the sample are shown to agree more strongly that pre–registration student nurses are encouraged to reflect on their clinical experiences. Explanation of this result is, however, difficult. There appears no logical explanation why such a significant result should have occurred. Explanation may be as Polit and Hungler (1991) relate that:

> there always remains the possibility that the obtained relationships may result from chance. (p.567)

Further exploration of the topic will, however, be conducted at later points in the research.

Generally there are more significant results pertaining to context variables. For example, respondents with cohort sizes of 40–59 and 60–79 are seen to be in less agreement that regular account is taken of students' learning styles in teaching sessions in their institutions' pre–registration nurse education programmes. It was shown also that significant results were obtained with regard to those with class size of on occasions 80–99 and over 100. These respondents felt that teaching adults was not different from teaching children and student–centred learning and teaching does not mean active learning. Explanations for these results may be inferred as relating to possible barriers to teaching and learning methods with regard to large students numbers. For example, those institutions with moderately high cohort numbers are less likely to be able to take account of individual student differences in terms of their learning styles. Also those institutions with on occasions relatively large class sizes are less likely conform to andragogical principles and incorporate active teaching and learning methods into their pre–registration nurse education programmes. However, again these tentative findings and explanations will be explored in more depth in later stages of the study.

There are also significant results pertaining to the context variables of academic level of pre–registration nurse education courses. For example, those institutions who offer certificate courses are more likely to agree that the principles of teaching adults are not different from those of teaching children. Explanation for this result may be, as discussed in the literature review, that traditional certificate level nurse education is associated with behavioural type teaching and learning philosophies and methodologies. These findings would therefore give some justification to the view that there is less incorporation of andragogical principles in institutions that are still conducting certificate level nurse education programmes.

The final significant result concerns those institutions which conduct diploma courses being more likely to agree that contract learning is used regularly in their institution. Again this may be due to using contract learning with large student group numbers as often typified by diploma level cohort and class sizes.

Factor analysis of the SAQ survey data

The final stage of data analysis of the SAQ survey is that of factor analysis. Polit and Hungler (1991) state that the main purpose of factor analysis is to reduce a set of variables into a smaller and more manageable set of measures. Factor analysis, therefore, explores interrelationships amongst variables and identifies which variables 'go together' as unified concepts. In the context of this study the aim of undertaking a factor analysis is therefore to examine whether there are any underlying and unifying dimensions in the ways respondents have responded to the attitude questionnaire.

The initial stage of the factor analysis was that of computing Spearman's correlations. The results of the Spearman's correlations are given in table 6.9. There are a number of significant results. For example, there is a highly significant correlation of responses between attitudes 4 and 5. Attitudes 4 and 5 relate to learning styles and learning preferences. There are also highly significant correlations between attitudes 10 and 11. Attitudes 10 and 11 relate to problem–solving and critical thinking skills. These examples may be seen to correspond to how the SAQ was initially devised. For instance, the questionnaire was structured around three key areas of student–centred learning which were seen to give rise to methods and beliefs about how they should be articulated in nurse education programmes. So, for example, problem–solving leads to valuing of critical thinking skills.

It may be seen that there is generally a high proportion of significant results. For example, all but two of the items (attitudes 1 and 6) are significantly correlated at less than 0.05 with one another. This suggests that they may constitute one or more factors and therefore further analysis is warranted.

Table 6.9
Spearman's correlation of attitudes 1-11

Att	1	2	3	4	5	6	7	8	9	10	11
Att 1	1.0000	-.581	.0295	0.203	-.0022	-.340	.200	-.909	.0682	.1055	.0159
Att 2	-.0581	1.0000	.1555	.1265	.1007	.1034	.3822**	.1312	.3454*	.4454*	.2432
Att 3	.0295	.1550	1.0000	.3194*	.2753*	.0762	.0032	.4406**	.3067*	.2873*	.4404**
Att 4	.0203	.1265	.3194*	1.0000	.7367**	.1995	-.0372	.4144**	.1676	.0883	.2065
Att 5	-.0022	.1007	.2753*	.7367**	1.000	.0507	.0422	.5078**	.1625	.2051	.2716
Att 6	-.340	.1034	.0762	.1995	.0507	1.0000	.0469	.1549	.1315	.0558	.0008
Att 7	.0200	.3822**	.0032	- .0372	.0422	.0469	1.0000	.1110	.3027*	.2448	.0827
Att 8	-.0909	.1312	.4406**	.4144**	.5078**	.1549	.1110	1.0000	.4210**	.4059**	.4602**
Att 9	.0682	.3454*	.3067*	.1676	.1625	.1315	.3027*	.4210**	1.0000	.6965**	.5481**
Att 10	.1055	.4454**	.2873*	.0883	.2051	.0558	.2448	.4059**	.6965**	1.0000	.5598**
Att 11	.0159	.2432	.4404**	.2065	.2716*	-.0008	.0827	.4602**	.5481**	.5598**	1.0000

1 - tailed significance: * - .01 ** - .001

The usual procedures of factor analysis as described by Kim and Mueller (1976) were subsequently undertaken. Table 6.10 gives the final factor analysis statistics.

Table 6.10
Rotated factor matrix

Att	Factor 1	Factor 2	Factor 3	Factor 4
Att 1	.02014	-.01270	-.09110	.93445
Att 2	.01587	.73502	.16714	-.04276
Att 3	.01587	.28547	-.40153	.16043
Att 4	.86483	.01141	.21755	.07049
Att 5	.87176	.02919	.07026	.04005
Att 6	.22013	.06524	.73269	-.08508
Att 7	-.16119	.66623	.35687	.24223
Att 8	.65878	.22205	-.13214	-.30304
Att 9	.21393	.78438	-.22125	-.02375
Att 10	.20667	.66686	-.21884	-.10060
Att 11	.41169	.46587	-.42134	-.25203

In general the meaning of a factor is determined by the items which load most highly on it. Kim and Mueller (1976) report that variables which correlate less than 0.4 with a factor should be omitted as these account for relatively small variances. Using this rule the following items may be seen to constitute each of the four factors identified in analysis of the SAQ data.

Factor 1

Attitude 5 is strongly correlated (.87176) with factor 1 and relates to regular account being taken of students' learning styles in the institution's pre–registration nurse education course.

Attitude 4 is correlated at .86483 and relates to regular account being taken of students' learning preferences in the institution's pre–registration nurse education course.

Attitude 8 is correlated at .65878 and relates to nurse teachers negotiating with students with regard to teaching and learning methods they use.

Attitude 11 is least strongly correlated (.41169) and relates to valuing critical thinking skills as an outcome of pre–registration nurse education courses.

Factor 2

Attitude 9 is strongly positively correlated (.78438) and relates to student nurses being encouraged to reflect on their clinical experiences.

Attitude 2 is positively correlated at .73502 and relates to self–directed learning as an important feature of student–centred learning and teaching.

Attitude 10 is positively correlated at .66686 and relates to problem–solving as an important feature of student–centred learning and teaching.

Attitude 7 is positively correlated at .66623 and relates to active learning as an important feature of student–centred learning and teaching.

Attitude 11 is least strongly positively correlated at .46587 and relates to valuing critical thinking skills as an outcome of pre–registration nurse education.

Factor 3

Attitude 6 is strongly positively correlated (.73269) to factor 3 and relates to the regular use of contract learning in the institution's pre–registration nurse education course.

Attitude 11 is negatively correlated (–.42134) and relates critical thinking as an important outcome of student–centred learning and teaching.

Attitude 3 is also negatively correlated (–.40153) and relates to self–directed study skills being taught in the institution's pre–registration nurse education course.

Factor 4

In contrast to the other factors there is only one item that is positively correlated with the factor. Attitude 1 has the strongest correlation of all the attitudes and is .93445. Attitude one relates to the principles of teaching adults being different from those of teaching children.

Summary of the factor analysis of the SAQ survey data

The main purpose of factor analysis of the SAQ was, as described earlier, to identify whether a conceptual framework exists in ways respondents scored their responses to the SAQ. It can be seen that two major factors have emerged. The first of these factors strongly unifies together taking account of learning styles, learning preferences and negotiation regarding teaching and learning. Weakly related is critical thinking as a valued educational outcome of nurse education. It is therefore argued that the major underlying concept of this factor is taking account of individual differences. It can be further argued that this concept is pivotal to the overall aim of this study which is to examine the interrelationships between student–centred teaching and learning and patient–centred care. For example, in the literature reviewed, individuality was identified as being of central importance in the articulation of patient–centred care through use of the nursing process.

The second major factor identified can be seen to relate to the importance of reflection on clinical practice and how student–centred learning is defined. This factor corresponds to major features of student–centred learning identified in the literature review. For example, self–directed, active and problem–solving learning were identified as key features of how student–centred learning is defined and articulated in nurse education. The factor analysis, however, a gives a further dimension to this definition though the addition of reflective learning on nursing practice.

Factors 3 and 4 may be seen to be significantly less important in terms of the amounts of variance they account for. Factor 3 has use of contract learning positively correlated and factor 4 teaching adults as being different from teaching children. Whilst there is substantially less evidence of the importance of these factors, it could be argued that underpinning concepts are valuing negotiation in teaching and learning, and acknowledgement that there are distinct differences to be considered when teaching adults as against teaching children. Valuing negotiation and andragogical principles in nurse education are therefore the underpinning concepts of factors 3 and 4.

Nurse teacher interviews

As described in previous chapters the next stage of data collection involved conducting a series of in–depth interviews with nurse teachers. A pilot study was conducted (n=5) prior to a main study (n=15). The nurse teacher sample was obtained from 20 different educational institutions in England offering pre–registration nurse education programmes.

Criteria for choosing of the interview sample is as described in chapter 5. However to recap, institutions selected to participate were chosen if they had obtained either low, medium low, medium, medium high or high scores in the attitude survey. A range of institutions offering differing academic levels of pre–registration courses also formed part of selection processes. For example, it was hoped to include institutions offering pre–registration courses at degree, diploma or pre–diploma level.

Nurse teacher interview sample details

An interview sample of nurse teacher for both the pilot study and main study was obtained from institutions representing the full range of SAQ scores. It was possible also to interview nurse teachers who had direct involvement with diploma and degree level pre–registration courses. It was not possible to find interviewees who had current involvement with pre–diploma courses. However, a number of those interviewed had past and, in some cases, recent past experience of teaching pre–diploma student nurses.

Respondents of the total interview sample were found as with the SAQ survey sample to comprise mainly of females (n=17). However, the majority of the interview sample were younger than the SAQ survey sample. For example, those in the interview sample were in the majority aged 30–39 years (n=11). There were similar characteristics in terms of how long the interviewees had been qualified as a nurse teacher, with the majority being qualified over ten years (n=8). There was one non–nurse teacher in sample and, as with the attitude survey sample, some non–qualified nurse teachers (n=4). Positions interviewees held within the educational institutions were again different from the SAQ survey sample as the majority were at nurse teacher (n=6) or senior lecturer grades (n=6). This may be compared to respondents of the SAQ survey who were found to fall into the senior educational management category. Appendix 4 gives details of the nurse teacher interview sample.

In conclusion whilst there are differences between the attitude survey sample and the interview sample, in its entirety the characteristics of the interview sample conform with achieving the aims of this stage of the research.

Nurse teacher interview data analysis

As described in previous chapters, main focuses of data analysis are identifying themes, categories and meaning units in the data. The major themes and categories of the main interview study are given in figure 6.1.

Also described in previous chapters is the fact that the lowest unit of data analysis was that of identifying meaning units which were ascribed to data categories. The final stage of data analysis was attributing a descriptive phrase to each individual or groups of meaning units. These were then tabulated. Each table therefore represents a data category with attributed properties of categories as given by the nurse teachers interviewed. The following section will examine each of the categories and their ascribed properties.

Theme one Learning theories as applied to nurse education
Category Definitions of student–centred learning and teaching

It is shown that a key belief is that students are responsible for their own learning and identifying their own learning needs. For example one respondent remarked:

21/5 2/11–12
They (students) are constantly reminded -they are working for themselves and they aren't going to be spoon fed.

(It should be noted for this and subsequent quotations that numbers in the left hand column are respondents' codes, and page and line numbers of the quotation.)

Other key areas are student opportunities for choice and negotiation in the learning process. These are similar concepts to those identified in the factor analysis of the SAQ data. In this analysis it has been shown that taking account of individual differences and learning needs is a key concept, along with teachers negotiating with students with regard to the teaching and learning methods used.

Taking account of individual differences is also shown to be important for the nurse teachers interviewed so students' different needs and wants are taken in account and teaching is tailored in respect of individuals' prior learning. For example, it was said to be important by one respondent to:

59/9 1/1–2
Find out what students already know and how they want to develop.

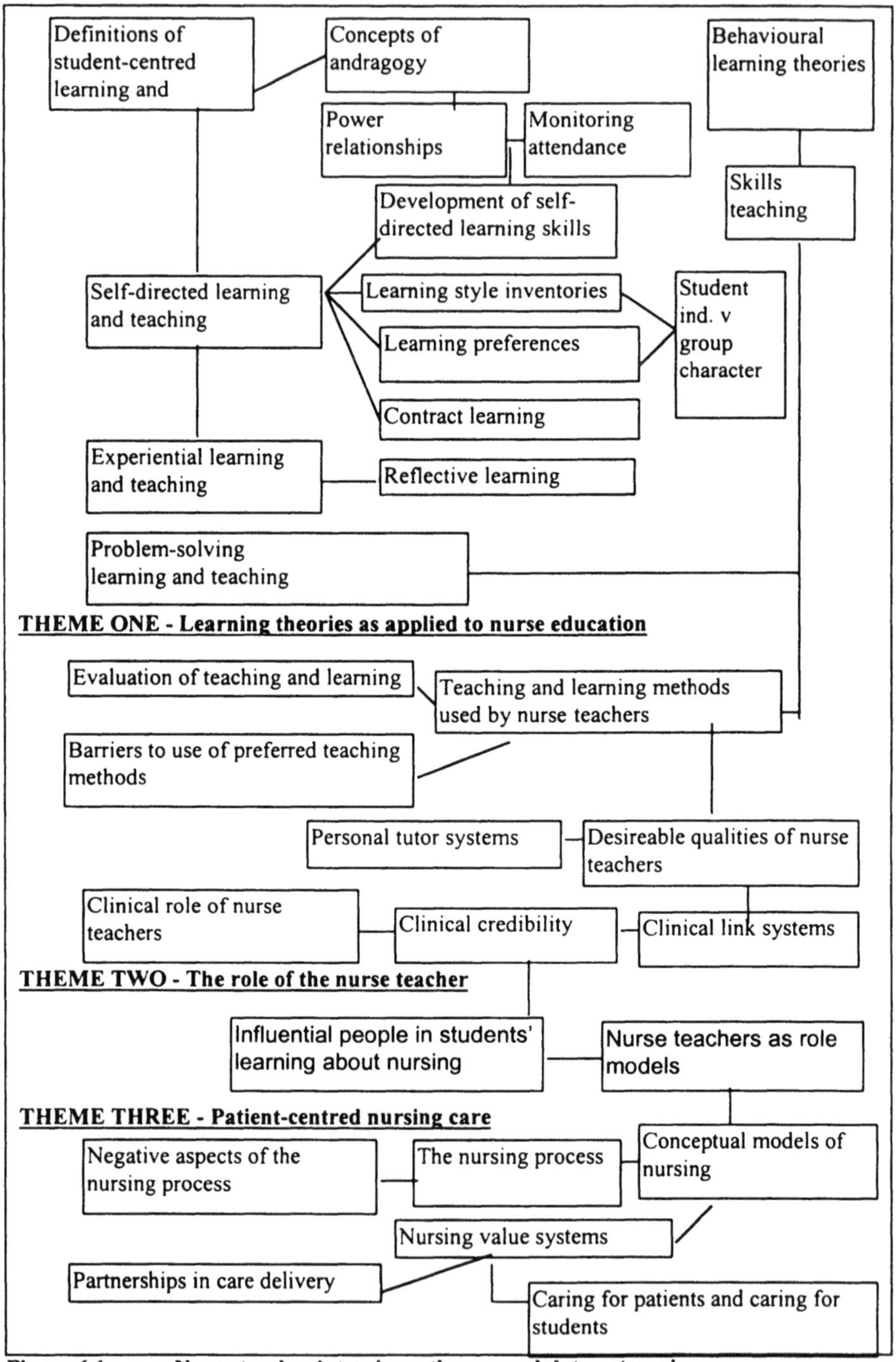

Figure 6.1 **Nurse teacher interviews, themes and data categories**

These majority views can be compared with a minority view who see student–centredness as being teacher–directed, with student–centred sessions being described as structured learning experiences. Two respondents' remarks also demonstrate a possible blurring between definitions of student–centred teaching and learning and concepts of andragogy. For example, it was said that student–centred learning should not be equated with immaturity and student–centredness is about treating students as adults. Finally one respondent found student–centred learning difficult to define and another that it is becoming popular dogma but was not being applied correctly. It was said by this respondent that:

> 78/3 1/2–4
> Student–centredness has become a bit of a bandwagon with some people. A lot of the time students are just left to work on their own.

Table 6.11

Definitions given of student–centred learning and teaching (n=12)

Properties:

1 Students taking responsibility for their own learning. 6 responses
2 Choice and negotiation in the learning process. 6 responses
3 Students identifying their own needs. 6 responses
4 Students being central. 4 responses
5 The teacher is a facilitator giving some information before students go and seek further information themselves. 3 responses
6 Enabling learning. 3 responses
7 Guidance and support for students. 2 responses
8 Facilitating students to learn in ways best suited to them. 2 responses
9 Having empathy with students through shared experiences. 2 responses
10 Student–centredness is being directed in some way, a student–centred session is a structured session where students are given guidelines to what is expected of them. 2 responses
11 The teacher finding out what students already know and how they want to develop. 1 response
12 Students have different need and wants. 1 response
13 Treating people as adults. 1 response
14 Certain teaching methods make the learning process student–centred. 1 response
15 SCLT has become a band–waggon with some people. 1 response
16 SCLT doesn't equate to immaturity. 1 response
17 SCLT is difficult to define. 1 response

Theme one	learning theories as applied to nurse education
Category	self–directed learning and teaching

Table 6.12 displays the properties attributed to self–directed learning and teaching. It can be seen that this category has the largest number of meaning units ascribed to it thereby making it the subject which the interviewees commented about most. However, it can be shown that the general trend of responses is consistent towards a belief that self–directed learning is an important aspect of student–centred learning and teaching theory. This may be compared to the general consensus view which was demonstrated in analysis of the SAQ survey when the statement pertaining to self–directed learning and teaching had high agreement scores.

Table 6.12
Self–directed learning and teaching (n=17)

Properties:

1 At the beginning students need to be given some basic facts and a framework for learning. 7 responses
2 Students don't know what to learn about and how to use SD study time effectively. 3 responses
3 SDL time can be seen as an excuse for lecturers not to do any work. 3 responses
4 SDLT is defined as students going out and finding information for themselves and working at their own pace. 3 responses
5 Students need support and guidance from lecturers when undertaking SDL. 3 responses
6 SDL is of more value when they are further on into the course and when they have some basic knowledge about the subject area. 2 responses
7 The tutor's role is giving framework for learning. 2 responses
8 Students initially need to be guided and directed as they start to develop SDL skills. 2 responses
9 Some students are not ready to undertake SDL where as others particularly A Level students are. 2 responses
10 SDL makes students feel insecure and lost because they lack basic understanding of the subject area and they are not used to this style of teaching. 2 responses
11 We don't take account of individual learning preferences and don't treat students as adult learners. 2 responses
12 SDL makes students more responsible for and autonomous in their learning and encourages independent thinking. 2 responses
13 Students cannot identify their own needs. 1 response
14 Students think lecturers don't respond to their needs. 1 response
15 In post–reg more SDL should be undertaken by students but they are still too reliant on lecturers. 1 response
16 I find defining SDL is difficult. 1 response
17 I expect students to come prepared for tutorials. 1 response
18 Monitoring open learning is difficult. 1 response
19 Sometimes we need to do lecturers and the very SD students think we are opting out. 1 response

Table 6.12 cont:

Properties: cont

20 Students have time to discuss what the SDL topic means for them and to what breadth and depth the subject area needs to studied at. 1 response
21 Students need to see SDL in a meaningful way and get feedback on their studies. 1 response
22 You cannot change attitudes through SDL this needs to be done through classroom teaching. 1 response
23 We have stopped using directed study as it was being over–used. 1 response
24 SDL means it's the responsibility of students to do the work and not for tutors to give information. 1 response
25 People are not self–motivated all the time. 1 response
26 SDL if done properly takes a lot more time than lectures. 1 response
27 Students still expect lectures and work to be given to them. 1 response
28 I am developing the use of work–sheets in the biological sciences. 1 response
29 There is a strong emphasis on SD study in our course. 1 response

General notions which can be identified in analysis of perceptions of self–directed learning and teaching are that students need some basic introduction to a study area before effective self–directed learning can occur. For example, one respondent said:

> 22/15 1/10–11
> They (students) need something concrete to start off with. I think teaching is about getting them off the ground.

A lack of basic understanding of a subject area was seen as a major barrier to effective self–directed learning by a number of respondents. For example, one nurse teacher remarked:

> 81/12 6/27–29
> Students are saying I would love to go and do something but I don't know what to learn.

There can be seen to be some degree of conflict with the point made earlier regarding the category pertaining to definitions of student–centred learning and teaching. In this category it has been identified that a key feature of student–centred learning and teaching is that students need to identify their own learning needs. This would mean that a basic understanding of the subject area is a prerequisite to identification of learning needs.

The role of nurse teachers in facilitating self–directed learning and teaching is also identified as being crucial. Guiding and supporting along, with adequate feedback to students, is said to be of great importance. For example, the possible student nurse experience of self–directed learning is described by one nurse teacher as follows:

86/14 1/19–21
It's not like teaching that has gone before. They (students) get quite insecure and say I don't know what I'm doing – tell me what to do.

However, whether or not this role is adequately fulfilled by nurse teachers is shown as being debatable. For instance it was said by one respondent that:

2/7 2/69–70
I think it can be an excuse for staff not doing any work.

Generally benefits of self–directed learning are seen as enabling students to be autonomous in meeting their own learning needs. However, also identified is the fact that effective self–directed learning hinges on self–motivation and re–orientation of student expectation away from use of directive, information–giving type teaching methods.

Theme one	learning theories as applied to nurse education
Category	development of self–directed learning skills

Development of self–directed learning skills is addressed in table 6.13. It is shown a large majority of those interviewed see self–directed learning skills as being addressed in study skills teaching. Some, however, do identify study skills teaching as being part of a self–development theme. For example, one interviewee said:

59/9 1/36–37
We've got it in theme one, personal development, which is about self–awareness.

The nature of the study skills course described varied. For instance, whilst a respondent said:

78/3 2/15–16
There's a study skills course in the CFP

another identified that:

90/4 2/27–28
It's usually a day's workshop at the beginning of the course.

Finally another interviewee said:

81/12 3/14–15
We look at that really with the study skills session....but again that's only a 2 hour session.

Table 6.13
Development of self–directed learning skills (n=15)

Properties:

1 Study skills (SS) sessions are done in an early part of the course. 6 responses
2 SS includes for example literature searching, note taking, referencing and creative writing but not sure if that's teaching SDL skills. 3 responses
3 SDL skills feature as part of a self–development theme. 2 responses
4 We use SS packages. 2 responses
5 SS should be taught at the beginning of the course. 1 response
6 Students lack SS when they start the course so I feel there should be a SS module at the beginning of the course. 1 response
7 The SS component of our course is only a 2hour session. 1 response
8 We only facilitate SDL through the use of profiling. 1 response
9 The teacher starts off the SDL process and may be part of that is teaching SDL skills. 1 response
10 Once students have developed SDL skills their capacity to learn increases. 1 response
11 There is a section in the library devoted to SDL skills. 1 response
12 SDL sessions means this is where you start to sort out your own learning skills 1 response
13 SDL skills are very important. 1 response
14 In SS we identify the level of academic study required. 1 response

It can therefore be concluded that whilst self–directed learning skills are valued by the nurse teachers interviewed, there is no uniform approach to how these are developed. For example, whilst some courses offer study skills modules others merely offer a single session on the subject.

These findings again correspond reasonably well with the SAQ survey findings where there was 53.947% strong agreement and 34.210% agreement that self–directed learning skills are taught in the institution's pre–registration nurse education course. 5.262% of the SAQ survey respondents disagreed that self–directed learning skills were taught. These disagreement scores may be compared with the remark made by one respondent who said:

> 85/17 2/21–23
> I've also felt when they start some of them (students) are very lacking in study skills. I've always advocated there should be an actual module on this.

However, it would seem generally from results of the SAQ survey and the nurse teacher interviews that lack of teaching regarding development self–directed learning skills is not the central issue. The issue would appear to be the amount of time spent on development of self–directed learning skills and the effectiveness of this teaching may be debatable. Also development of self–directed learning skills are a valued part of education outcomes of pre–registration nurse education courses.

Theme one learning theories as applied to nurse education
Category learning style inventories

Table 6.14 displays the properties of learning style inventories as given by the nurse teacher interview sample. As discussed in the review of the literature, it can be demonstrated that learning styles have links with self–directed learning and teaching. For example, in considering how to develop self–directed learning skills it is thought to be important to take account of differences in the ways individuals learn. Learning style inventories are one way these differences can be identified. However, with the SAQ survey statement pertaining to the utilisation of learning style inventories, whilst there were 51.314% agreement scores, the scores generally grouped around the middle value scores, with 21.052% disagreeing with the statement. The data obtained from the nurse teacher interviews do not diverge from the findings of the SAQ survey. The highest number of comments in this category demonstrate that learning style inventories are not generally utilised in respondents' institutions. Where learning styles profiles are compiled it is part of a self–awareness theme as against a deliberate attempt to tailor teaching methods to preferred ways of learning. For example, one respondent said:

81/12 6/8–9
We take no notice of learning styles because with a group of 129 to accommodate everybodies' learning style is difficult.

Table 6.14
Learning style inventories (n=10)

Properties:
1 As far as I am aware we don't do the learning style profiles of our students. 4 responses
2 Learning style inventories of students are done as part of the teaching study skills, individual needs and drives and communication skills. 3 responses
3 Personal teachers help students develop their own learning style through profiling and the use of personal learning journals. 2 responses
4 It's difficult to take account of the variety of learning styles. 2 responses
5 If learning style inventories are done the time and resources must be made available allow account to be taken of them. 2 responses
6 I don't know what learning style inventories are. 2 responses
7 Identifying individual learning styles are about fostering self–awareness. 1 response
8 Learning styles are about the way an individual learns best. 1 response
9 I don't ask students what their learning style is. 1 response
10 Undergraduate students don't have a wide range of learning styles. 1 response

Finally in conducting the interviews it was noticed that instruments available for measuring learning styles were rarely mentioned. Generally an impression was obtained that for a number of those interviewed there was little understanding of what was implied by learning style inventories and there was a blurring between this concept and that of learning preferences.

Theme one learning theories as applied to nurse education
Category learning preferences

The results of the SAQ survey regarding learning preferences gives a similar picture to the data obtained for learning style inventories. There was, for example, no clear agreement that learning preferences were taken into account of in the institutions surveyed. However, in the section related to Chi–Square analysis of comparisons of attitude with cohort size a significant result was obtained in that less regard is taken of learning preferences with institutions with cohort sizes of 40 to 79. These findings may be compared with those of the factor analysis where the major factor which emerged out of the SAQ survey data was the importance of taking regard of learning preferences.

Table 6.15 shows that learning preferences are said to be generally taken into account by the nurse teachers interviewed. As concluded in the factor analysis, negotiation is identified as a key feature of taking account of individual learning preferences. This is seen as being articulated through negotiations with students about how teaching sessions are structured. For example one respondent said that:

34/10 4/21–23
I think the majority of teachers would be open to some negotiation at the beginning of a session.

and another that:

88/1 2/14
If students say they want a lecture I think I would do that.

Whether or not learning preferences are taken into account is seen as being monitored by course evaluation strategies. (Evaluation of teaching and learning is the focus of a separate category analysed later in this theme.)

Difficulties, however, of having regard for individual preferences are seen as being related to individual teaching styles and being influenced by such things as inflexible time–tabling. Also identified by one nurse teacher is that not all students preferred a negotiated approach. It was said by this respondent that:

34/10 4/24–26
It's my experience that for the majority of the time they (students) are quite happy to accept what you are going to give them.

Table 6.15
Learning preferences (n=11)

Properties:

1 The majority of teachers are be open to negotiation at the beginning of a session/course to how the topic is going to be taught. 5 responses
2 I think I take account of students' learning preferences. 2 responses
3 The effectiveness of taking account of learning preferences is monitored through evaluation systems. 2 responses
4 Individual groups differ in how they like to learn and in their ability to negotiate. 2 responses
5 Taking account of students' learning preferences is difficult because of the size of the groups. 2 responses
6 Students would like to have more negotiations regarding how they learn. 1 response
7 Some lecturers would negotiate with students, some would not. 1 response
8 We don't always allow for individual learning preferences because the evaluation system makes us work in retrospect. 1 response
9 We assess students' individual needs through use of a questionnaire. 1 response
10 We negotiate our teaching methods to stop students becoming bored. 1 response
11 Teachers trained in the last 10 years are able to adapt their teaching style to fit with group learning preferences. 1 response
12 Students need to be prepared before–hand if a session content is going to be decided by them. 1 response
13 Taking account of students' learning preferences is difficult because of the size of the groups. 1 response
14 Students are quite happy to accept how the teacher decides to teach. 1 response
15 It is difficult to give the students the freedom to learn in the way they would like to because of timetabling problems. 1 response
16 Students want more clinical experience. 1 response

However, some of those interviewed felt that learning preferences could only be accommodated in terms of group preferences as against individual preferences. For example, one respondent remarked:

81/12 1/27–28
The difficulty is when you've got a group of 100 trying to get consensus amongst them.

As there were a relatively large number of comments focussing on group versus individual teaching and learning preferences, separate data analysis of this subject was conducted. These results are presented in the following section.

Theme one learning theories as applied to nurse education
Category student individuality versus group characteristics

Table 6.16
Student individuality versus group characteristics (n=10)

Properties:

1 Because of the large numbers of students in groups only group learning needs can be catered for. 7 responses
2 Often I do not know the students names because of the large numbers of student I deal with. I sometimes get around this my calling them pet names. 5 responses
3 Individual differences are recognised but it is difficult to take account of them. 1 response
4 Some students say the College doesn't care for them. 1 response
5 The group get penalised if individuals in the group do anything wrong. 1 response
6 Individuals get treated as individuals in tutorials. 1 response
7 There is an analogy regarding treating a group of students in a similar way to treating a ward of patients the emphasis should be on the people. 1 response
8 There is an analogy regarding assessing a student's needs in a similar way to assessing patient's needs. 1 response
9 I try and call students by their christian names. 1 response
10 We build in group interactions to help personal development. 1 response

Table 6.16 shows that a substantial number of respondents identify the fact that large groups being taught makes it difficult to take account of individual learning preferences. However, paying attention to learning preferences is not the sole issue. It is seen by number of those interviewed that taking cognizance of learning preferences related to being valued as an individual. For example, one nurse teacher interviewed commented:

> 70/11 8/1–4
> Being in such large numbers I do feel, apart from personal students contact, a lot of the time they (students) don't feel valued as individuals. They feel part of the herd.

Manifestations of treating students as individuals are seen as being related to, for example, whether or not individual students are known by name. The difficulties of this were, however, commented on by one interviewee who said:

> 60/20 1/21–25
> When I had a group of 80 after a few weeks yes I did (know students' names) but it was a real effort. With 250 no chance. I wouldn't know some of them if they walked past me in the street.

whereas another respondent remarked:

> 34/10 3/23
> The other way I get around it is calling them by a pet name.

Caring for students was also a focal issue with some respondents comparing how students are cared for with how patients are cared for. For example, when comparing treating students as individuals one respondent said:

70/11 7/29–30
I suppose you assess students' needs as you assess patients' needs.

It can therefore be generally concluded from these findings that caring for students in terms of taking account of individual needs and differences can be compared to caring for patients through taking account of individual needs and differences. Institutional systems designed to meet individual student needs are discussed further in the role of the nurse teacher theme when personal tutor systems are analysed.

Theme one learning theories as applied to nurse education
Category contract learning

One approach that can be taken to individualise teaching in order to meet the individual learning needs of students was identified in the review of the literature as being through the use of contract learning. However, in analysis of the SAQ survey data the statement regarding contract learning was identified as one which generally had the highest disagreement scores. Significant results were also obtained with regard to the context variable of diploma level pre–registration education. Respondents from these institutions were less likely to agree that contract learning is regularly used in their institution's pre–registration programme. It may therefore be inferred from these results that contract learning is not in general use and specifically is not used extensively in diploma level courses.

Table 6.17, however, shows a number of teachers interviewed purporting to use learning contracts. For example, one respondent commented:

89/2 2/35–36
I've had learning contracts with some of my students who've failed their exams.

Table 6.17
Contract learning (n=14)

Properties:

1 Learning contracts are used with students who have an identified weakness and have failed an examination or assignment. 4 responses
2 Using learning contracts is time consuming. 3 responses
3 Learning contracts are used in informal ways. 2 responses
4 Learning contracts are used on the EN conversion course. 2 responses
5 Learning contracts are used with the child branch students. 2 responses
6 I think contract learning is beneficial as it is something that addresses individual student needs. 2 responses

Table 6.17 cont:

Properties: cont

7 Contract learning is not appropriate for use in teaching the biological sciences. 1 response

8 Learning contracts have no place with students who know nothing. 1 response

9 I couldn't use contract learning with the amount of students I teach. 1 response

10 Learning contracts are artificial. 1 response

11 Learning contracts are not used in our College. 1 response

12 Learning contracts are used with registered practitioners in terms of theory components of their course. 1 response

13 Learning contracts involve a lot of paper work to start off with. 1 response

14 Learning contracts are very labour intensive. 1 response

15 Contract learning is used in the college. 1 response

16 Learning contracts identify the parameters of a relationship. 1 response

17 Contract learning isn't always successful and I think it's to do with maturity. 1 response

18 I use contracts for students first clinical experience as it helps them to know what they should be achieving. response

19 Although students should have learning contracts with their personal tutors it's very much a paper exercise. 1 response

Others identified how learning contracts could be seen by students as a way of individualising or personalising the learning process. For example, one nurse teacher interviewed said:

> 62/20 2/25–26
> I personally find it (contract learning) very beneficial. Students see it as something just for them.

Some of those interviewed also commented that there are particular courses where the use learning contracts is more appropriate. However, generally contract learning was seen to be used on an informal basis and dependent on teacher preferences. Moreover a number of the nurse teachers interviewed identified some of the inherent difficulties of using contract learning. For example, one respondent commenting on these disadvantages said:

> 59/10 2/23–24
> It's (contract learning) a paper exercise and too time–consuming

In conclusion, it can be seen that contract learning is not in wide–spread use although it is seen as a way of personalising learning needs.

Theme one learning theories as applied to nurse education
Category experiential learning and teaching

The next major category of student–centred learning and teaching is that of experiential learning. In analysis of the SAQ survey data it was found that generally high agreement scores were obtained with the statement that student–centred learning means active learning. In the factor analysis it was also shown that active learning was a dimension of how student–centred learning was defined by the respondents. However, it was shown in Chi–square analysis that there was a significant difference in the responses of institutions with have class sizes on occasions of 80 to over 100 students.

Table 6.18 generally reflects the findings of the SAQ survey that experiential learning and teaching are seen as being important in pre–registration nurse education. However, experiential learning is defined by the majority of those interviewed as active learning in classroom type situations and away from clinical areas. For example, whilst two respondent mentioned that experiential learning occurred through reflection on practice no one one mentioned it in direct relationship to gaining clinical experience. The majority saw it as developing nursing skills through teacher–contrived classroom type learning situations. For example, one respondent gave an example of how when:

62/20 2/12–14
Doing eating and drinking we get them (students) to feed one another jelly whilst they are in bed.

Table 6.18
Experiential learning and teaching (n=17)

Properties:
1 Students learn through experience. 3 responses
2 ELT is used by tutors in getting students to appreciate possible experiences patient may have. 3 responses
3 Lectures include ELT. 3 responses
4 Lectures use role play methods. 3 responses
5 ELT is used in communication skills teaching. 3 responses
6 A lot students don't want to get involved in activity learning they prefer lectures. 3 responses
7 ELT is not student–centred because the activity is initiated by the tutor. 2 responses
8 ELT in classroom activities helps students to apply theory to practice. 2 responses
9 ELT is part of student–centred learning because they are learning for themselves. 2 responses
10 ELT methods are used more with mental health branch students. 2 responses

Table 6.18 cont:

Properties: cont

11 ELT can be tiring and stressful. 2 responses
12 ELT is really important. 2 response
13 I don't use ELT much as I haven't got the skills to use it. 2 responses
14 Teachers are not forced to use ELT methods. 1 response
15 Teachers should create situations where students are active. 1 response
16 ELT methods are not suitable for teaching the biological sciences. 1 response
17 In ELT learning occurs through reflection on experience. 1 response
18 I want to include more ELT through involving practical laboratory work. 1 response
19 The students are asked how much ELT should be included in sessions. 1 response
20 Because of the large numbers of students on the course there isn't time to use all the students' clinical experiences to identify what has been learnt. 1 response
21 Recently qualified teachers use activity learning. 1 response
22 EL is not appropriate for structured sessions. 1 response
23 If it is well managed students can learn through ELT. 1 response
24 Students often use ELT methods in their own presentations. 1 response
25 We try and balance lectures with seminar work on a 1:2 ratio. 1 response

This type of activity was seen as a way of bridging the gap between what is taught and what is practised. In addition certain nursing specialities, namely mental health nursing and certain subject areas, were seen as more amenable to experiential teaching and learning methods. For example, one interviewee remarked that:

> 70/11 2/19–21
> We do a lot of experiential learning in communication skills.

Whereas another said:

> 88/1 1/12–13
> In the subject area I teach (biological sciences) it's difficult to use experiential learning methods.

However, experiential learning and teaching were also seen by a number of those interviewed to include activities given to students in lectures. For example, one nurse teacher who taught biological sciences said:

> 88/1 1/15–16
> I try and involve the students by asking plenty of questions for example.

It is also identified that students do not always like these types of teaching and learning methods and it is sometimes a tiring and stressful way to learn. For instance it was said by one interviewee that:

> 81/12 2/12–13
> If it's activity learning a lot of them (students) just don't want to know. They like lectures.

Finally teaching skills required for effective use of experiential methods are also identified as being important.

In conclusion, whilst it can be seen that the interviews conducted give greater depth to understanding how experiential teaching and learning is perceived, the responses are in broad agreement with the scores obtained in the SAQ survey.

Theme one	learning theories as applied to nurse education
Category	reflective learning

Table 6.19
Reflective learning (n=13)

Properties:

1 Reflection is associated with evaluation of clinical practice. 8 responses
2 Students are encouraged to write about their experiences in diaries or learning journals. 7 responses
3 Students experiences are used in a critical incident format to analyse issues. 5 responses
4 Reflective practice is introduced early on in the course. 3 responses
5 Reflective sessions are more effective with older or post–registration students. 3 responses
6 Reflection is valued in the College. 2 responses
7 There is no way of ensuring that students keep a reflective diary in an effective fashion. 2 responses
8 Reflective sessions are included in an implicit rather than explicit ways. 2 responses
9 Reflective sessions are done informally. 2 responses
10 Reflection is done in groups. 1 response
11 Reflective skills are used in the course. 1 response
12 Reflective practice is going to be introduced soon in the CFP. 1 response
13 Students have time in the day given over to personal reflection. 1 response
14 Reflection is student–centred. 1 response
15 The reflective diary is not an assessed piece of work it is used to demonstrate attendance. 1 response
16 Older people are more confident in analysing situations. 1 response

As discussed in the review of the literature reflective learning can be seen as learning from experience. This may be compared with learning through experience. In an essentially practical profession it is clear that both these forms of learning are of extreme importance.

The importance of reflective learning is demonstrated in analysis of results of the SAQ survey, where it was found that there was generally strong agreement that student nurses are encouraged to reflect on their clinical experiences. However, it was shown in analysis of the independent variable of sex the male respondents in the attitude survey were less likely to agree that pre–registration student nurses are encouraged to reflect on their clinical experiences. Initial analysis of this category of data therefore examined the interview transcriptions of the males' nurse teachers. No insights could be found from this analysis of why males in the SAQ survey should give significantly different responses from females in the sample. The three male nurse teachers gave positive responses to questions relating to students reflecting on clinical practice. It is therefore concluded as previously hypothesised that this finding of the SAQ data occurred by chance.

The results of the nurse teacher interviews displayed in table 6.19 give further evidence of the importance attributed to reflection on clinical practice. For example, one respondent commented that:

> 70/11 3/8–9
> When they (students) come back off placement they always have a reflection on practice session.

The way reflection skills were developed was identified by a number of those interviewed. For instance:

> 79/16 2/20–22
> The learning journal is really good for this, getting them (students) to look at things, reflect on things.

Learning journals or reflective diaries are also described as being of use in identifying critical instances which could be used as a focus for group discussions. However, it was also noted that it was difficult to ensure that all students actually did keep diaries. Finally it was considered by some respondents that true reflection on nursing practice was an ability only associated with mature or experienced nurses.

Theme one learning theories as applied to nurse education
Category problem–solving learning and teaching

It was shown in analysis of the SAQ survey data that responses to the statement pertaining to problem–solving learning and teaching as a feature of student–centred theory gave the highest and most unequivocal score of any of the attitude statements. The interview data given in table 6.20, however, demonstrates that problem–solving activities are generally perceived by the nurse teachers interviewed as relating to methods of delivering nursing care. For instance, one respondent remarked that:

> 81/12 9/1–2
> Most of our exercises are designed in theory to use a problem–solving approach. Mostly nursing problems.

The importance of problem–solving skills in nursing practice was also highlighted by the non–nurse teacher interviewed who commented that:

> 29/13 5/6–9
> If you're giving a saline drip you need to know about it. It isn't just taking it and putting it up like an idiot. They are meant to take some responsibility and know what they are doing.

However, a small minority of those interviewed did view problem–solving in a more general context and talked about how problem–solving skills can be developed. For example, it was identified that students need to work out the solutions to problems themselves. It was suggested by one nurse teacher that it could be developed thus:

> 21/5 1/15–16
> As the tutor I just take a guiding brief and put in the odd word here or push them a little so it actually comes from them.

In conclusion, it can deduced that problem–solving skills are identified as being of importance in nursing practice. However, the ways in which these skills are developed in nurse education programmes would appear not to conform to a structured approach and not to feature as part of general teaching and learning strategies.

Theme one	learning theories as applied to nurse education
Category	concepts of andragogy

How the concept of andragogy is perceived by the nurse teachers interviewed constitutes one of the final threads in the learning theories theme. It was shown in analysis of the SAQ survey data that there were strong agreement scores with the statement that the principles of teaching adults are different from those of teaching children. It may therefore be concluded that there is evidence that the respondents surveyed have strong positive beliefs regarding the general concept of andragogy.

Table 6.20
Problem–solving learning and teaching (n=13)

Properties:

1 PSLT is associated with nursing practice and the use of the nursing process. 6 responses
2 PPLT can be developed through allowing students to work out the answers to questions themselves. 3 responses
3 PSS are taught in our course. 2 responses
4 Teaching PPS is a developmental process. 2 responses
5 PSS are developed through the use of a reflective journal and practical experiences. 2 responses
6 PS approaches are student–centred. 1 response
7 How PS activities are used depends on the topic area. 1 response
8 PS may be seen in a similar light to hypothesis testing. 1 response
9 PS is addressed in a scientific approaches section of the course. 1 response
10 Students can PS and help other students learn. 1 response
11 In practice nurses need to be able reason things out. 1 response
12 PS can be encouraged when teaching certain nursing skills. 1 response
13 PSS are taught in the CFP. 1 response
14 PSS are needed by students. 1 response

It was also shown, however, in analysis of the SAQ survey data that those respondents whose institutions are still conducting pre–Project 2000 certificate level course were significantly less likely to agree that the principles of teaching adults are different from those of teaching children. As concluded earlier these results conform with the general conclusions of the literature review. So, for example, traditional nurse training (pre–Project 2000 certificate level courses) are demonstrated to be teacher–centred and pedagogical in orientation. In contrast, progressive nurse education is described as being student–centred and andragogical in orientation (Hurst 1985).

A central focus of the interview data displayed in table 6.21 is the fact that andragogy is seen as being treating students with respect. This may be compared to concepts explored in the literature review relating to andragogy as not merely concerned with age difference but also with status differences. However, whether or not these status differences are respected is doubted by some of those interviewed. For example, one interviewee commented that:

> 34/10 4/1–2
> Teaching children is different to teaching adults but you wouldn't think so sometimes.

Other andragogical principles were also identified by those interviewed. For example, it was shown in the literature review that andragogy implies that adults have a range of life experiences to which teachers can relate new learning. This principle is articulated by one nurse teacher interviewed who said:

88/1 1/5–7

They (students) bring their own life experiences with them and the teacher must build upon this knowledge.

Adult learners were also identified by some of those interviewed as being more independent and self–directed in their learning. For example, one respondent commented that:

89/2 1/5–7

Student–centred learning is used with children but children need more direction. They can't identify what they need to learn.

This is, however, in direct contrast with some of the findings regarding the self–directed learning and teaching category, where it was said that some basic comprehension of the subject area being studied is necessary before effective self–directed learning can occur. It can be seen that there is conflict in the data regarding the relationship between andragogy and student–centred learning. For example, nearly equal numbers differed in their beliefs that student–centredness is the same as andragogy. However, in as much as a separate category of data has emerged it would appear that some differences can be identified. It would appear from a majority point of view of those interviewed that andragogy is valued more as a belief system or ideology. This may be compared with student–centred learning and teaching, which has been shown in previous categories as being defined in terms of a learning theory.

Table 6.21
Concepts of andragogy (n=12)

Properties:

1 Andragogy is about respecting people. 4 responses
2 Students are not always treated as adult. 3 responses
3 Student–centred methods of teaching can be used both with children and adults. 3 responses
4 Andragogy is not the same as student–centreness. 3 responses
5 Andragogy and student–centreness have shared principles. 2 responses
6 The teacher should build upon the previous experiences of life adults have. 2 responses
7 Andragogy means adult students are more independent and self–directed in their learning. 2 responses
8 Children need more direction in their learning as they can't identify their own learning needs. 1 response
9 Andragogy is an exploratory way of learning which students find anxiety provoking and confusing. 1 response
10 Andragogy should mean students have structured teaching which incorporates some student choice. 1 response
11 Older people have more confidence in voicing their opinions. 1 response

Table 6.21 cont:

Properties: cont

12 People generally don't always act in an adult fashion. 1 response
13 Andragogy isn't just about age differences. 1 response
14 Younger adults need more focus and support. 1 response
15 Student–centredness doesn't embrace the humanistic aspects of andragogy. 1 response

Theme one learning theories as applied to nurse education
Category power relationships

Respectful egalitarian–type relationships can be seen as pivotal in analysis of concepts of andragogy. This category extends the analysis further through examination of the concept of power in nurse teacher/student nurse relationships. It is shown in table 6.22 that student nurses are believed to have a good deal of power in respect of meeting their learning needs. However, it is thought that nurse teachers have the most power. For example one nurse teacher interviewed said:

78/3 1/25–26
Ultimately the power base is still with the tutors and the college.

Empowering students in their learning was also identified as being difficult by a number of those interviewed. For instance one interviewee remarked:

2/7 4/24–25
A lot of the time they don't want to be empowered.

and another said:

78/3 1/29–31
Even ward sisters revert into a student mode. It's like they have gone back to school. That's still how it's perceived. So the power is seen to lie with the tutors.

Table 6.22
Power relationships (n=9)

Properties:

1 Whilst students have a lot of power and can negotiate with teachers it's still the teachers who are in control. 3 responses
2 It's hard work empowering students as a lot of the time they prefer to be passive. 2 responses
3 Students don't feel they are equal to lecturers. 2 responses
4 Students are powerful in the University because they are consumers of a degree programme. 1 response

Table 6.22 cont:

Properties: cont

5 Even experienced nurses when they are students revert back into a passive mode. 1 response

6 As nursing students they are not powerful. 1 response

7 There are bureaucratic constraints to moving power to a more equal basis. 1 response

8 We haven't empowered our Project 2000 diploma students. 1 response

9 A lot of tutors have problems dealing with students on an equal basis. 1 response

10 Some staff think I am too responsive to students and therefore they are too powerful. 1 response

11 Because I have more knowledge about nursing this influences equality in the student/teacher relationship. 1 response

Theme one	student–centred learning and teaching
Category	monitoring attendance

An example of how power is articulated in pre–registration nurse education programmes was identified by a number of interviewees as being through monitoring attendance (see table 6.23). So, for example, one of those interviewed said:

> 24/18 2/22–23
> Lectures are there and we've got this notion that students should attend.

Another interviewee said that student attendance was monitored by teachers and so:

> 86/14 6/8–10
> We have to call a register. Is that student–centred? I'm not an idiot. They sign other people in. You've destroyed the idea of student–centredness as soon as you walk in the classroom.

However, the majority of those interviewed whilst, agreeing that attendance was monitored in their institution, said, for example:

> 34/10 3/3–4
> It's fine for students not to go to lectures if they can demonstrate prior learning in the subject area.

Student attendance is further discussed in the category related to barriers to teaching and learning and in regard of statutory requirements governing pre–registration nurse education. However, generally it can be concluded that the interviewees' institutions appear to have differing policies regarding compulsory attendance, with some taking a more liberal view than others.

Table 6.23
Monitoring attendance (n=8)

Properties:

1 Non–attendance at certain sessions can be facilitated but there is a ceiling on how many sessions students can miss. 4 responses
2 In the College there is a belief students should be attending all sessions. 2 responses
3 Students have to attend lectures unless they can demonstrate proficiency in the subject. 2 responses
4 Often students don't attend and reasons for non–attendance are not given. 2 responses
5 Some students are conscientious and attend all the sessions. 1 response
6 We use registers of attendance and these destroy the idea of student–centreness. 1 response
7 Large class sizes mean an increase in absenteeism. 1 response
8 Some students attend lectures because that's the best way for them to learn. 1 response

Theme one learning theories as applied to nurse education
Category behavioural learning theories

The subject area of this category changes the focus of analysis and addresses manifestations of behaviourist learning theories in pre–registration nurse education. Such theories are shown in the literature review as being in direct contrast to student–centred learning theories and andragogical beliefs. It was also shown in the literature review that behaviourist theories of learning are not overtly dominant in nurse education philosophical belief systems, the dominant theory being student–centred cognitivist type theory. The comparatively small number of responses relating to this category displayed in table 6.24 may be viewed as giving further credence to the lack of popularity of behaviourist type learning theories. However, the agreed focus of comments made in this category is in favour of a balanced approach. For example, one nurse teacher said:

7/6 4/23–24
I would be sad if the curriculum, the philosophical approach wasn't a balanced one.

Also an eclectic approach to how individual students are seen to learn was viewed as being important by another interviewee who commented:

85/17 3/10–11
I think there are a lot of theories but I don't think we can identify one student a particularly theory applies to.

However, another respondent commented on a point explored earlier that basic knowledge of a subject area is a prerequisite of student–centred learning activities. This interviewee said:

> 81/12 8/1–3
> To me there are just some things you've got to know and then develop an understanding of it afterwards. To me this is rote learning.

The implication is therefore that behaviourist theory needs to be applied in initial learning of a subject area.

Also identified is the fact that nursing process and associated problem–solving activities in essence a behavioural approach. This may be compared with some of the conclusions drawn from findings of the literature review, where it was shown that there is an inherent tension with the humanistic philosophy underpinning the concept of person as viewed in approaches to care delivery. This humanistic individualistic philosophy may be contrasted with the rational, logical and objective features of the system of care delivery featured in a nursing process approach. Essentially it is seen that the nursing process utilises behaviourist type theory as a basis for care delivery but is underpinned by humanistic type philosophical beliefs.

Table 6.24
Behavioural learning theories (n=6)

Properties:

1 The curriculum should be a balanced one and be informed by a number of learning theories. 4 responses
2 Rote learning is not appropriate in a nursing course. 1 response
3 Human being are complex and one theory of learning cannot account for all these differences. 1 response
4 Problem–solving utilises a behavioural approach. 1 response
5 Behavioural objectives are used in skills development. 1 response
6 Teachers set learning objectives in our College. 1 response
7 We have to be directive and teacher–centred when students don't know what they want. 1 response
8 There are certain areas of knowledge students must know and initial rote learning of this knowledge is appropriate. 1 response

Theme one	learning theories as applied to nurse education
Category	skills teaching

Finally it is shown that learning about nursing practice is also seen as being largely governed by behaviourist theory. For instance one interviewee said:

7/6 48/30–32
Putting a student in a clinical area to undertake certain objectives. They're behavioural objectives essentially. So the approach which is taken to gain a skill is a behavioural one.

The subject of learning nursing skills was focused on by a relatively large number of those interviewed and therefore is the central feature of the following category in this theme.

The importance of teaching certain nursing skills prior to students going into clinical areas is seen as important by the majority of those interviewed (see table 6.25). One interviewee went so far to say:

90/4 3/31–33
Unless we address it (skills acquisition) in a safe environment then some schools run the risk of being exposed to malpractice in some form.

Safe practice by students was therefore seen to be of prime importance. However also identified was the fact that:

32/8 5/7–8
The students were feeling very insecure about were they seeing enough in the clinical areas.

Generally an impression is gained that skills teaching in clinical areas is the ideal but for a variety of reasons this is not occurring and therefore a number of institutions are undertaking this type of teaching now, or planning to do so in the future, in the form of skills workshops. However, it can be seen that skills needed for nursing practice are not solely defined in terms of psycho–motor skills. A number mentioned developing skills needed for effective communication and interpersonal relationship attributes. For example one teacher said:

32/8 4/33–34
The communication and counselling sections are all skills based. It's all practice using videos.

Table 6.25
Skills teaching (n=11)

Properties:

1 Nursing tasks such as for example TPR's are taught in the classroom. 4 responses
2 Students feel more confident going into clinical areas knowing they have practised certain practical skills. 3 responses
3 The college is going to have a skills laboratory soon. 3 responses
4 Students have skills workshops 2 response
5 Interpersonal skills are taught in. the classroom. 2 responses
6 We teach nursing skills in the clinical areas whenever we can. 1 response

Table 6.25 cont:

Properties: cont

7 We have got rid of the practical room and now we haven't got the facilities to teach lifting and handling to the students. 1 response
8 We have gone to the extreme and don't do any skills training at all. 1 response
9 The students didn't feel they were getting enough skills training. 1 response
10 When student undertake a practice teaching session most of them choose to teach a skill. 1 response
11 Students should be taught and practice certain skills before they go out into clinical practice. 1 response
12 In children's nursing it is important that skills are adapted to the age of the child. 1 response
13 Students need supervision when they are doing physical tasks. 1 response
14 Clinical staff don't always have the time to teach students how to do nursing tasks. 1 response
15 Unless students can practice nursing tasks in the safe environment of the College some Colleges run the risk of having a malpractice case being brought against them. 1 response
16 Skills training is undertaken by clinical or teaching staff or those who see themselves as clinically credible. 1 response

Finally a key issue for one interviewee was the fact that where such teaching took place was not a major issue. The major issue for this nurse teacher was who teaches the skills and whether the person is clinical competent. This issue can be seen to be related to the role of the nurse teacher, which is the central area of exploration in the next major theme of this analysis.

Theme two the role of the nurse teacher
Category teaching and learning methods used by nurse teachers

The second theme identified in the data analysis of the nurse teacher interviews is role of nurse teachers. Whilst the previous theme focused upon teaching and learning principles and methods, this theme is devoted to looking at how nurse teachers are influenced by these learning theories when teaching pre–registration nursing students. This theme is an implicit rather than explicit part of the data analysis. For example, few direct questions were posed pertaining to the theme. A substantial amount of the data has therefore been obtained from examples and illustrations the nurse teachers gave when asked about learning theories.

Table 6.26 gives the learning and teaching methods purported to be used by the interviewees. The two meaning units accruing the majority of comments are those of two seemingly diametrically opposed teaching methods. For example, a number of the interviewees commented in a similar vein that:

86/14 2/14–16
There's nothing wrong with didactic teaching. I know everyone is talking about andragogical approaches but sometimes the students say, "give me some facts".

As shown in the literature review, didactic lecture–type teaching methods are most commonly associated with behaviourist type learning theory.

However, a number of those interviewed said small group or one to one tutorials are frequently used teaching methods. For instance, one nurse teacher interviewed remarked that:

59/9 1/20–21
We get them to question things in private one to one tutorials.

Table 6.26
Teaching and learning methods used by nurse teachers (n=14)

Properties:

1 There is time allocated for small group tutorials. 7 responses
2 Often students appreciate lectures because they want the straight forward delivery of facts. 7 responses
3 Students don't enjoy group work. 4 responses
4 Using a variety of teaching methods is best. 4 responses
5 Students are exposed to a number of different teaching methods including workshops, self–directed learning packs, seminars, lectures and gaming. 4 responses
6 The choice of teaching method depends on the subject being taught. 3 responses
7 A main lecture and then small group teaching is the approach used in our College. 2 responses
8 Humorous and enjoyable sessions helps learning. 2 responses
9 Group work is useful as it helps students to think for themselves and develops trust and rapport within the group. 2 responses
10 Use of a traditional lectures is the standard practice in the College, student participation in these lectures in minimal. 2 responses
11 A lot of lectures involve dictation of information to the students especially when we started Project 2000. 2 responses
12 The use of a traditional lectures was the standard practice in the College when the new curriculum was introduced it is, however, different now. 1 response
13 We have gone from being too didactic to being too laissez–faire. 1 response
14 Passive learning allows the students to have a rest. 1 response
15 The method of teaching depends on the group preferences. 1 response
16 Nursing studies are taught mainly in seminar groups. 1 response
17 Student participation can happen in lectures. 1 response
18 Lectures are mostly a waste of time. 1 response
19 Lectures are easy to do well unlike group work. 1 response
20 Students enjoy group work. 1 response
21 The majority of the course should be taught using group work. 1 response

Personal exploration of a subject area in this fashion is commonly associated with student–centred cognitivist learning theory.

A number of those interviewed, however, said using a variety of teaching methods which also incorporate humour and are enjoyable is best. Also teaching methods used depend sometimes on the subject being taught and student–group preferences. Moreover teaching methods which fall within the general remit of each learning theory were also identified as having associated problems. For example, lecture–type methods were seen as being disliked by a number of those interviewed. The non–nurse teacher interviewed said, for instance:

> 29/13 2/1–2
> It's standard practice. You stand up and talk and nobody says anything. I've scrapped that. It's ridiculous.

At the same time a number of those interviewed said that group work was a useful teaching method and helped students to develop independent thinking skills. As a teaching method it was also said by some to be enjoyed by students. However, a corresponding number of those interviewed commented, for instance:

> 79/16 2/6–7
> They (students) are pleased when they haven't got to do any group work.

It can be concluded from this section that of the teaching methods used by those interviewed no one method can be identified as being more effective. Therefore both behaviourist and student–centred cognitivist type theories can be seen to be an influence in the teaching methods used in pre–registration nurse education. The articulation of methods which broadly match the tenets of each theory can, however, be seen to have associated problems. The effectiveness of teaching and learning methods is the focus of the following category of this theme.

Theme two the role of the nurse teacher
Category evaluation of teaching and learning

A relatively large number of the nurse teachers interviewed discussed how teaching and learning evaluation strategies are utilised in their institutions. As shown in table 6.27 a major point made, however, was that no matter what strategy is deployed it is difficult to be certain if effective learning has taken place.

A number of those interviewed, however, did refer to a product–type teaching evaluation which is normally associated with behavioural type learning theories. For example, one interviewee said evaluation depended upon:

> 89/2 4/22–24
> Whether your objectives have been met, their (student) objectives have been met.

In a similar vein others said assessment results were another way to measure whether teaching and learning had been effective. For instance, it was identified by one of those interviewed that:

> 90/4 2/31–33
> Only through assessments can you ensure learning has taken place.

However, a corresponding number of those interviewed also referred to more process–centred evaluation methods, student comments on the effectiveness of teaching and learning methods being one way this type of evaluation may be conducted. For example, when referring to evaluation of clinical practice a nurse teacher interviewed said:

> 2/7 2/54–55
> We have a formal sit–down session when they come back to evaluate it.

Table 6.27
Evaluation of teaching and learning (n=12)

Properties:

1 You can't really be sure if effective learning has taken place. 4 responses
2 Assessments and assignments can show if effective learning has taken place. 3 responses
3 Groupwork can be evaluated by student feedback. 2 responses
4 Changes to the course as a result of student evaluations happens in retrospect. 1 response
5 We ask students which sessions they have found most useful. 1 response
6 We have informal meetings with students where course evaluation is addressed. 1 response
7 Evaluation is concerned with whether or not the objectives have been met. 1 response
8 Course evaluation is done through the use of questionnaires but I don't think they address the real issues as the return rate is poor. 1 response
9 We need to respond if students say they are not getting what they want. 1 response
10 Course evaluation occurs at the end of each period of time in college. 1 response
11 My instincts tell me when my teaching has been effective. 1 response
12 Students can't see the point of completing evaluation forms as they feel no one takes any notice of what they say. 1 response
13 Clinical practice is evaluated through a formal session when they return to the University. 1 response
14 Evaluation of the course, particularly the clinical component is seen as being important. 1 response
15 The College responses to students' evaluations of the course. 1 response

Generally it was felt by some interviewees that whilst students' views were elicited regarding teaching effectiveness, their relative significance as against the more product–type evaluation measures was under–valued. For example, one interviewee remarked that:

86/14 8/28–29
Students say to me "I can't see the point in doing these evaluations because nobody takes any notice " .

This comment can be seen to have inter–relationships with the previously discussed category of power relationships in nurse teacher–student nurse interactions. Thus whilst students appear to have power through having a significant input into curriculum evaluation, the actuality may be that student comments are not taken into account. Therefore student power to effect change over their learning conditions is negated.

Evaluation of teaching and learning strategies may also be seen to relate to the final categories in this theme regarding barriers to preferred methods of teaching. For example, student evaluations may indicate that changes are needed but because of some of the more inflexible aspects of curriculum delivery such changes are not possible.

Theme two the role of the nurse teacher
Category barriers to use of preferred teaching and learning methods

Table 6.28 displays the barriers to the use of preferred teaching and learning methods as identified by the nurse teachers interviewed. It is seen that there are seven areas identified as having an influence on how pre–registration nursing students are taught. The first of these refers to resource issues, with major factors being identified as inadequate classroom accommodation. This may be seen to interrelate to the second factor, which is large groups which often have to be split up for teaching sessions. A number of those interviewed said these problems accrued as a direct consequence of implementing Project 2000 diploma type courses. For example, introduction of pre–registration diploma courses has been coupled with a dramatic increase in sizes of student groups. However, there has been little difference in provision of accommodation for teaching pre–diploma students. (Pre–diploma cohorts to Registered Nurse training courses are usually smaller, with more frequent intakes, and they spend less time in the classroom and more time in clinical areas.)

This general picture is also demonstrated in analysis of the SAQ data where over half of respondents (52.631%) reported cohort sizes of over 80 and over one fifth (22.368%) reported cohort sizes of over 120. Also analysis of the SAQ survey data showed that 28.947% of institutions reported that their pre–registration class size may on occasions be over 100 and 34.210% that their institution's class size on occasions is 40–79 students.

Table 6.28
Barriers to the use of preferred teaching and learning methods (n=17)

Responses:
Resources:
1 Inadequate classrooms. 11 responses
2 Lack of time is a barrier. 4 responses
3 Inadequate library facilities is a barrier. 3 responses
4 Lack of equipment and chairs for classrooms. 3 responses
5 Resources are a barrier. 2 responses
6 Financial constraints are a barrier. 2 responses
7 The College is multi–sited. 1 response
Class size:
1 The size of the groups. 7 responses
2 The average group size is manageable providing we split the groups up. 7 responses
3 Mental health and child branch numbers are small which can sometimes cause a problem. 2 responses
4 The number of groups. 1 response
Teacher resources:
1 Teachers who's teaching is at times inadequate and do not use student–centred teaching methods. 3 responses
2 Not enough teachers is a barrier. 2 responses
3 The age of the tutor and how long they have been teaching. 2 responses
4 Attitudes of tutors to other tutors. 1 response
5 Tutors who are clinically competent and those who are not. 1 response
6 Teachers who are not used to teaching at diploma level. 1 response
7 Not enough teachers who can teach certain subject areas. 1 response
8 Inexperience and lack of confidence in teachers. 1 response
The curriculum:
1 It's a prescribed document with an inflexible approach to it's implementation. 4 responses
2 Nobody being sure what should be taught. 1 response
3 Short placements. 1 response
Professional bodies:
1 The minimum number of theory and practice hours imposed by the ENB. 3 responses
2 Constrains imposed by the ENB. 3 responses
3 Constrained by the competencies. 1 response
Student expectations:
1 Students expecting to have didactic teaching. 2 responses
2 Domineering students who don't give quieter members of the group the chance to speak. 1 response
College regulations:
1. Constraints of the College regulations. 1 response

Those offering pre–registration nursing degree courses, whilst not governed by National Health Service regional manpower planning figures (as pre–registration nursing diploma course are), still identified large group numbers as being a barrier to use of certain teaching methods. However, reasons given here are that a number of higher educational institutions have increased student intake numbers as a result of financial considerations.

Inflexibility in terms of design of the curriculum, college polices and the influence of the statutory bodies governing nurse education are also identified as being barriers to preferred teaching methods. However, following resource issues and group size the next largest category was that related to teacher resources. A number of those interviewed saw inadequate teaching skills as being a problem, coupled with a shortage of teachers who had the appropriate clinical experience or theoretical knowledge to teach certain subjects. These issues will be analysed in greater depth in some of the following categories which pertain to the clinical dimension of nurse teacher's role.

Theme two	the role of the nurse teacher
Category	desirable qualities of nurse teachers

The category given in table 6.29 relates to qualities and attributes seen as being desirable for nurse teachers. As identified in a number of the categories previously analysed the nurse teacher's role was seen by a number of interviewees as being a facilitator of learning, a resource person or someone who has expert knowledge of a subject area. This generally fits with a cognitivist student–centred type model of the role of the nurse teacher. An example of this perspective is given in the following quotation when one of those interviewed said their primary function was:

20/19 1/2–1
Meeting individual student needs.

Table 6.29
Desirable qualities of nurse teachers (n=13)

Properties:

1 To be a facilitator of learning who supports and encourages students and gives them the freedom to learn. 7 responses
2 To be a resource person. 3 responses
3 To be an up–to–date expert and a giver of knowledge. 3 responses
4 Meeting individual student needs. 1 response
5 Teachers have a disciplinary role. 1 response
6 To be a friend to the student. 1 response

Theme two	the role of the nurse teacher
Category	personal tutor systems

How this type of role is accommodated against the previously described back–drop of inadequate resources, large student groups and difficulties in taking account of different student learning styles and learning preferences is addressed in the following data category.

A large majority of nurse teachers identified that their institution had an effective personal tutor system. Table 6.30 demonstrates that it is through such systems that needs of individual students are seen as being catered for. For instance, one interviewee said:

> 52/9 2/16–17
> If they have a problem as an individual it gets dealt with – they have a personal tutor.

The caring nature of these personal tutor/student relationship was also seen as being important by a number of the nurse teachers interviewed. For example, one of those interviewed said:

> 70/11 8/9–10
> I would hope from a personal tutor point of view they don't feel uncared for.

A personal tutor system based on a new student group being allocated to a number of different nurse teachers appeared to be the predominant model described. A small number, however, identified a system whereby one tutor acted as personal tutor to cohort group. This system was identified by the non–nurse teacher interviewed as being an unsatisfactory system. For example, it was said by this interviewee that:

> 29/13 6/7–9
> Thirty seven people with a cohort leader is a joke. I would scrap that and have personal tutors.

Finally a number of those interviewed commented that student counselling services were also available to address individual student needs and problems.

Table 6.30
Personal tutor systems (n=12)

Properties:

1 We have an effective personal tutor system whereby personal tutors can give both academic and pastoral support to students. 6 responses
2 Students are encouraged to share and reflect on their experiences with their personal tutor. 3 responses
3 Individual tutorials are done by students' personal tutors. 3 responses
4 The College has or has access to a student counselling service. 3 responses
5 Once I have got to know my personal tutees I care about them. I enjoy this humanistic part of my job. 3 responses

Table 6.30 cont:

Properties: cont

6 Students are encouraged to go to their personal tutor. 2 responses
7 Personal tutors can get to know their students quite well and therefore can treat them as individuals. 2 responses
8 It is alright if students don't go and see their personal tutors. 2 responses
9 The cohort tutor acts as a personal tutor for students as a group. 2 responses
10 Initially students don't have any choice in who their personal tutor is. Although later on they can change if students want to. 2 responses
11 The College's student charter says students must have a named personal tutor. 1 response
12 A minority of tutors don't support their personal tutees enough. 1 response
13 I have more than 20 personal tutees which is regarded as the maximum a tutor should have in our College. 1 response
14 I would only give my home phone number to certain of my personal tutees. 1 response
15 Non–nurse teachers should be allowed to be personal tutors. 1 response

Theme two	the role of the nurse teacher
Category	the clinical role of the nurse teacher

The clinical role of nurse teachers was identified by a number of those interviewed as an important but problematic area. Major features of this role are depicted in table 6.31. In the table it is demonstrated that models of clinical teaching are given by a number of the nurse teachers as being a supportive role as against one of conducting formal clinical teaching sessions. For instance, it was said by one interviewee that:

59/9 4/14–15
I don't really work with them. I just visit them to support them.

Generally, however, the clinical facet of the nurse teachers' role was seen as being difficult to address adequately. For example, one of the interviewees commented that:

86/14 8/2
The system has not enabled me to do what I would like.

Reasons for this appeared to be related in part to teaching resource issues. For example, a nurse teacher said clinical teaching was possible but:

22/15 2/17
It is time consuming. For us it's a killer.

Others also commented that clinical teaching was ineffective and needed to be addressed in their institution in a structured fashion. Formal strategies for addressing the clinical teaching role of nurse teachers are addressed in the following category which is related to clinical link systems.

Table 6.31
The clinical role of the nurse teachers (n=12)

Properties:

1 Lecturers do clinical visits to support students but don't necessarily work with the students. 6 responses
2 The College needs to address the issue of lecturers working in clinical areas as clinical teaching is ineffective. 4 responses
3 The University has a system where lecturers can work in clinical areas with students but this doesn't happen as often as lecturers and students would like. 3 responses
4 Placement visits are labour intensive and time consuming. 3 responses
5 Nurse teachers are given the time to go into practice areas to maintain their own competence. 2 responses
6 Students don't always like to be visited in clinical areas. They think they have done something wrong when we do. 1 response
7 Students enjoy seeing their tutors in clinical areas. 1 response
8 Diploma students resent undergraduate students being visited by their lecturers as diploma student lecturers don't visit them. 1 response
9 The College no longer has anyone who undertakes a clinical teacher role. 1 response

Theme two the role of the nurse teacher
Category clinical link systems

Table 6.32 addresses comments made by the nurse teachers regarding clinical link systems. It is shown that the majority of those interviewed said their education establishment had a clinical link system. Generally this was described as a system whereby nurse teachers had designated clinical areas to visit. For example, one nurse teacher interviewed commented:

79/16 5/8
All the clinical areas have a link teacher.

However, number of those interviewed saw such systems as being problematic. Another interviewee commented:

89/2 6/39–41
It's a very sore point you're touching on right now in this college. I started here in July and ever since I've being begging (for a link ward). I've always had link wards.

and another said:

86/14 7/35–37
I get angry when I talk about this. At the moment myself and another guy, the two of us link with the whole of the district general hospital.

How nurse teachers' clinical link roles are defined is variable. Some thought it was up to the individual teacher to negotiate their role with the clinical area. Whilst others saw the role as directly related to the student education being conducted in the clinical area. For instance, one of those interviewed equated clinical link systems with clinical teaching and said:

22/15 3/16–17
The College students resent that we (University lecturers) come out because the College tutors don't.

Table 6.32
Clinical link systems (n=12)

Properties:

1 The College has a clinical link system. 2 responses
2 Although the College has a clinical link system I haven't got a clinical link at present so I don't know how effective it is. 1 response
3 I really want a clinical link ward but I have been unable to get one. 1 response
4 Clinical links are important. 1 response
5 The clinical link system we have is a little territorial. 1 response
6 It is up to the individual to negotiate the link teacher role. 1 response
7 We are just implementing a clinical link system. 1 response
8 There are not enough teachers to have an effective clinical link system. 1 response
9 We have a clinical link system but it doesn't work very well mainly because of time factors. 1 response
10 The College is not committed to clinical practice and therefore the clinical link system doesn't work in a meaningful way. 1 response
11 Developing effective clinical link systems are difficult for Higher Education establishments. 1 response

An added implication of this comment is that University lecturers are seen as having a greater clinical teaching focus than those teaching diploma students.

Finally it can be concluded from analysis of the interview data that none of those interviewed associated clinical link systems with maintaining their own clinical competence. However, the issue of clinical competence did feature in the interviews and is discussed in the following category.

Theme two the role of the nurse teacher
Category clinical credibility

Table 6.33 displays the notions of clinical credibility described by the interviewees. Whilst clinical link systems are not seen in terms of maintaining clinical credibility, the majority of those interviewed did see maintaining clinical credibility as an important issue. A relatively large number said that they were able to undertake clinical practice. However, a number said that the way they undertook this practice was through:

62/20 5/13–14
Agency work, I do the odd Sunday morning to keep my hand in.

However, clinical credibility was seen as being more important than clinical competence for one of those interviewed, who remarked:

32/8 8/31–34
In fact there are very able tutors who are getting a bit rusty. When they go into the clinical area they will ask staff to show them. The students have no problem with that. They have difficulty when people are giving them naff information.

Table 6.33
Clinical credibility (n=11)

Properties:

1 I do some agency work partly so I am able to maintain my clinical competence. 5 responses
2 A number of nurse teachers in our institution work in the clinical areas regularly in order for them to maintain their clinical competence. 4 responses
3 Lecturer–practitioners that are employed in the College are clinically credible. 3 responses
4 Maintaining clinical credibility is important. 2 responses
5 It would take a lot of resources to enable me to become clinically credible again. 2 responses
6 Geographical divides between college and clinical areas makes it more difficult to go and practice on the ward areas. 1 response
7 I keep myself up–to–date by exhibiting students' work in health centres and doing staff preparation sessions. 1 response
8 I don't think it's possible for nurse teachers to maintain their clinical credibility. 1 response
9 Some nurse teachers are completely out of touch with realities of clinical practice. 1 response
10 Some nurse teachers are well know in the clinical areas and are part of the ward team. 1 response
11 I no longer think of myself as a nurse but as a teacher. 1 response

Also identified by some of those interviewed was the fact that a minority of nurse teachers are not clinically competent and that it was unrealistic to expect nurse teachers to be so. One interviewee commented:

> 62/20 5/35–36
> There are some (nurse teachers) who wouldn't know a patient if it hit them.

and another said:

> 59/9 4/17–18
> If you want me to become clinically credible you are going to have to let me go to a ward area where there aren't any students so I can reorientate myself.

The final issue that can be identified in this category is the importance of how students view nurse teachers with regard to learning about nursing practice. It was said by one interviewee that:

> 85/17 5/17–20
> I've worked with students who don't think you've worked on the wards. They are quite shocked when you say you've been a nurse.

Central to this comment is a definition of nurse teachers as role models for students learning about nursing practice which is the focus of the following category.

Theme two the role of the nurse teacher
Category nurse teachers as role models

The subject of this category may be seen as one of the central issues in this investigation. Table 6.34 gives perceptions of the interviewees regarding notions of nurse teachers acting as role models for students learning about nursing. Generally it may be concluded from analysis of data in the previous categories that it is difficult for nurse teachers to maintain regular clinical contact. In line with these conclusions, when asked about their position as a role model for students learning about nursing, it would appear that the majority of those interviewed did not rate themselves or their colleagues as being important in a practical, clinical context. For example, one of those interviewed said:

> 21/5 8/16–18
> It's not the same as being by the bedside and acting as a role model for them. I think they would find it very useful if they could see some of us in action.

However, others interviewed did see themselves acting as role models for students learning about nursing in a clinical context. Furthermore some identified themselves as acting as role models for students in a more indirect fashion and in classroom type situations. For example, an interviewee commented:

85/17 4/21–23
I think in what I say about patients. When I talk about patients or my experiences they (students) get an impression of me as a carer.

It may therefore be concluded that there is no consensus amongst those interviewed regarding whether nurse teachers act as role models for student nurses when they learn about nursing. As it is questionable that nurse teachers are seen as being central to how student nurses learn about nursing practice, other influential people on this process is the focus of the following category.

The final category in this theme pertains to who are seen by those interviewed as being influential in how student nurses learn about nursing. Table 6.35 gives the responses obtained. It can be seen that an the overwhelming majority identify clinical staff as being the most importance. For example, it was said by one interviewee that:

20/19 2/23–24
The qualified nurses are the most powerful (role models).

Table 6.34
Nurse teachers as role models (n=13)

Properties:
1 Nurse teachers are not role models but they would be if students saw them practising in clinical settings. 4 responses
2 I don't believe nurse teachers are role models for students. Clinical staff are. 3 responses
3 Because we can draw upon our clinical experiences students may see us as role models. 3 responses
4 Because I am seen in clinical practice by students I think I am a role model for them. 3 responses
5 Students think I'm out of touch with reality and don't know I've been a nurse. 2 responses
6 Nurse teacher need to have a good breadth of clinical experience before they become teachers. 1 response
7 Nurse teachers are role models when students are initially not having much clinical experience. 1 response
8 Personal tutors can be role models depending on the strength of the relationship. 1 response
9 Nurse teachers may act as teaching role models for students. 1 response
10 When I go out into practice I tell them when things are not good nursing practice. 1 response
11 Students don't object to tutors being a little out of date. What they object to is being given the incorrect information. 1 response
12 To act as a role model a nurse teacher has to be a good teacher. 1 response

Theme two the role of the nurse teacher
Category influential people in how students learn about about nursing

Others interviewed said that the student nurses' own peers were also influential. It was, for instance, said by another interviewee that student nurses learn about practice:

81/12 11/22–23
From each other, senior students helping junior students.

Perceptions of students learning about nursing from one another were seen in the review of the literature to be associated with traditional apprenticeship style nurse training. For example, Chandler (1991) describes how it is thought that the advent of diploma level training and integration of nurse training into higher education establishments will change the traditional socialisation processes of nurse training.

It would appear from findings of this study that there is some evidence that this is not the case. However, the subject will be addressed again in subsequent areas of data analysis when pre–registration student nurses' perceptions of who are influential when they learn about nursing will be analysed.

Table 6.35
Influential people in how students learn about nursing (n=18)

Properties:
1 Clinical staff. 18 responses
2 Peers and peers who have had some nursing experience. 5 responses
3 Nurse teacher can be influential if they have a good relationship with the students. 3 responses
4 Patients. 2 responses
5 Clinical supervisors or mentors. 2 responses
6 Joint appointment and clinically competent tutorial staff. 2 responses
7 I just hope they chose they role models wisely. 1 response
8 Sometimes students don't chose their role models wisely. 1 response
9 A number of different people . 1 response

It can be shown generally from results of this category that whilst clinical staff are seen as being the most influential, others are also seen as having influence. For example, patients and nurse teachers are identified as also being important.

Theme three patient–centred care
Category the nursing process

The final theme in this section addresses the delivery of patient–centred care or how clinical nursing practice is approached in the view of those interviewed. In contrast to previous data themes, data pertaining to this theme emerged in a explicit fashion from a number of direct questions in the interview schedule regarding personal values of nursing.

Table 6.36
The nursing process (n=9)

Properties:
The nursing process implies-

1 A systematic approach. 6 responses
2 Assessment, planning , implementation and evaluation. 4 responses
3 A framework for care. 2 responses
4 A problem–solving approach. 3 responses
5 The whole process of nursing. 1 response
6 Something not appropriate for health visiting practice. 1 response

It was shown in the review of the literature that use of the nursing process is advocated as a desirable way of delivering nursing care. Perceptions of the nursing process as an objective product–type system of care delivery is demonstrated in data presented in table 6.36. Most of those interviewed agreed that:

32/8 6/15–16
It's a logical systematic approach

They also identified it as a problem–solving approach which has assessment, planning, implementation and evaluation as key stages to care delivery.

Theme three patient–centred care
Category negative aspects of the nursing process

Analysis of data in this category pertains to the negative aspects of use of the nursing process. It is shown in table 6.37 that just under half of those interviewed felt that there were negative aspects of the nursing process. For example, one of interviewee thought that the way it was used in clinical practice was problematic and said:

21/5 6/22–24
This is just a lot of paper work for the sister to do. Let's reduce this to the minimum. Let's have a reductionist model. Let's have boxes to be ticked.

Whilst another commented that:

34/10 6/6–7
We have care plans in theory and care plans in practice.

This last comment also has direct relevance to the purported theory:practice divide in nursing, or what is taught in the educational establishment not being of relevance to what is practised in clinical areas.

Finally it was identified by some interviewees that the nursing process is an objective logical system. For example, it was said by one nurse teacher that:

22/15 3/1–2
I have problems with the nursing process because it requires students to evaluate against goals.

Generally the central importance of the nursing process as articulating the philosophical underpinning of nursing practice is debatable. Data analysis reveals that it is seen as a systematic method of delivering nursing care. For example, it was shown in the pilot study of the nurse teacher interviews that questions pertaining to the nursing process did not receive any responses regarding nursing value systems. However, some of the responses did refer to conceptual nursing models of care when asked about value systems pertaining to nursing practice.

Table 6.37
Negative aspects of the nursing process (n=9)

Properties:
1 The nursing process is poorly used in the clinical areas. 3 responses
2 Use of the nursing process was badly introduced in this country. 3 responses
3 Nurses do not understand how to use nursing process properly. 3 responses
4 The nursing process implies a lot of paper work. 2 responses
5 The nursing process is a product–orientated approach which requires evaluation against pre–determined goals. 2 responses
6 Patient assessment needs to be taught effectively as it the key to correct use of the nursing process. 1 response
7 Correct use of the nursing process is difficult because of a shortage of clinical staff. 1 response
8 The use of core care plans is undesirable. 1 response
9 Nursing care given is not evaluated properly. 1 response
10 Care plans done in the College sometimes are not the same as care plans found in practice. 1 response
11 The nursing process is viewed in a linear rather than cyclical way. 1 response

Conceptual models of nursing care are therefore a feature of the next data category.

Theme three	patient–centred care
Category	conceptual models of nursing

Table 6.38 gives the synthesised comments made by the nurse teachers regarding conceptual models of nursing care. It is shown that a number of interviewees thought they had their own personal conceptual model which informed their approach to patient care. For example, one nurse teacher remarked:

59/9 3/20–21
I've always had a nursing model that goes from your head to toes.

Other interviewees said that it was important that student nurses were introduced to a variety of conceptual models. For example, it was said by one interviewee that:

81/12 10/16–17
We look at how each author of a model utilises the nursing process for practice.

The data also demonstrate, as with the use of the nursing process, negative observations regarding the use of conceptual models. However, a key feature of this section of data analysis is the fact that conceptual models are used to frame the nursing process and to give its use a distinct philosophy. The major importance of conceptual models used is, in the words of one interviewee:

21/5 5/40–42
My whole thing is which one is going to address the individual needs. Where will one work and another not.

Table 6.38
Conceptual models of nursing (n=10)

Properties:
1 I've got my own model of nursing that I use in practice. 2 responses
2 Students are taught about models and how each model informs the use of the nursing process. 2 responses
3 I don't know anything about nursing models. 1 response
4 Everybody seems to use the same model where or not it's appropriate for the clinical area. 1 response
5 The models used needs to be appropriate for the particular clinical areas. 1 response
6 Models should frame the use of the nursing process. 1 response
7 I believe models are more important than the use of the nursing process. 1 response
8 I'm anti–models I find them limiting. 1 response

However, whilst it has been shown that conceptual models of care are generally felt to give a formalised philosophical basis for care, a further dimension to this subject can be identified. This added dimension shown at the beginning of the data category is the personal belief systems of those interviewed regarding nursing care. These personal value systems are examined in the following category.

Theme three patient–centred care
Category nursing value systems

The data displayed in table 6.39 demonstrates that the majority of those interviewed appear to have personal belief systems regarding nursing practice which is similar to that explored in the review of the literature or a humanistic orientation to care–giving. For example, one nurse teacher interviewed commented that:

> 24/18 3/33–34
> Caring is recognition of an individual. Their rights, their position in society, their humanness I suppose.

This comment also reveals the perceived affinity between the term caring and nursing which is further demonstrating in the following quotation when an interviewee remarked that:

> 79/16 3/25
> To me nursing is about caring.

Caring was also identified in terms of caring about the needs of individuals, their welfare and well–being.

These findings may be compared with earlier analysis of the interview data, where similar concepts were identified as being of importance in terms of student–centred learning and teaching. For example, a key issue in the factor analysis of the SAQ survey data was taking account of individual differences and needs. Similarly in analysis of the nurse teacher data on definitions of student–centred learning and teaching, learning styles, learning preferences and contract learning it was shown that concepts of individuality were thought to be important. Caring for students was also a central issue in the category pertaining to personal tutor systems.

It may, therefore, be concluded that there are a number of similar features regarding concepts of student–centred learning and teaching and patient–centred care. Individuality in addressing both student and patient needs appear to be key concepts. Also concepts of care are important in terms of being applied both to caring for students and caring for patients. Finally whilst in–depth exploration of how these finding relate to the published literature is the subject area of the following chapter of this study it can be general shown that the findings are in accord with conclusions drawn from the literature.

Table 6.39
Nursing value systems (n=11)

Properties:
Nursing should be about–

1 Recognising and valuing peoples' individuality and their humanness. 7 responses
2 Identifying patients' problems. 2 responses
3 Caring. 2 responses
4 Meeting patients' needs. 1 response
5 Putting the patient first. 1 response
6 Not just caring but about looking after the welfare and well–being of patients. 1 response

Table 6.39 cont:

Properties: cont

7 Patient–centredness. 1 response
8 Treating people with dignity. 1 response
9 Developing empathy and understanding for patients. 1 response

Theme three patient–centred care
Category partnerships in care delivery

Table 6.40 gives the responses of those interviewed regarding how patients are involved in decisions regarding their care. It can be seen that shared planning of care is dependent on attitudes of staff in different clinical areas. For example, one interviewee said:

90/4 4/21–23
It varies in clinical settings. In some settings it's not so. Providing the patient is breathing in and out that's OK.

whereas another said that:

32/8 6/27–29
We've got a co–ordinated care project going on. For the first time ever the patient discusses and signs to say they agree with all this.

There are also a number of comments relating to how patients' involvement in their care should be dependent on the attitudes of the individuals being cared for. For instance, one nurse teacher remarked:

21/5 6/8–13
Could be the patients don't want it to happen. You've got an old boy who says you're the nurse and I don't want to know. Or you're got some other person who's highly educated and wants to know their diagnosis. Individual wishes must be taken into consideration.

Generally, however, it can be seen from data in this category that those interviewed did not think patients were treated as equal partners in nurse/patient relationships. Therefore in a similar fashion to how nurse education is thought to be teacher–centred, patient care is thought to be nurse–centred.

Theme three patient–centred care
Category caring for patients and caring for students

Table 6.40
Partnerships in care delivery (n=11)

Properties:

1 Shared planning of care works well in some clinical areas. 3 responses
2 Nurses sometimes need to recognise that patients do not always want to share in decision–making regarding their care. 3 responses
3 Nurses still think they know best. 2 responses
4 Patients are not involved in planning their own care. 2 responses
5 Patients sometimes don't know enough of what is wrong with them to be true partners. 1 response
6 The nursing process restricts individual choice because the nurse decides the outcomes of care. 1 response
7 Patients are not treated as equal partners in the decisions regarding their nursing care. 1 response
8 Nurses have gone too far the other way and don't let parents opt of of caring. 1 response
9 Shared planning of care varies in clinical areas. 1 response
10 Nurse/patient relationships should be equal. 1 response
11 Patients are never asked how they want to be cared for. 1 response
12 Nursing is still nurse–centred. 1 response
13 Equal nurse/patient relationships are about negotiating the needs of the patient. 1 response

The final category of data analysis of the nurse teacher interviews addresses the pivotal question of the perceived relationships between caring for patients and caring for students (see table 6.41).

The nurse teachers thought generally that they were caring towards their students. This was seen as being because nurse teachers are nurses themselves. For example, some thought there had been a transfer of their caring role with patients to students. For instance, one interviewee remarked:

> 7/6 7/17–19
> One of the ways that I have got to grips with changing from a clinical role is in some ways I have just changed my client group.

However, the quality and quantity of caring for students was identified as being different from that given to patients. For example, it was said by one interviewee that:

> 85/17 5/1–2
> You might be over–caring for patients but not for students.

Generally, however, it is agreed by the majority of those interviewed that the concept of role imitation is important or the notion that if students are cared for by their teacher they will replicate this caring attitude in the delivery of patient care. For example, one nurse teacher said:

32/8 7/25–27
This student said (to me) "I think we are taught how to care because we have role models in the nurse teachers".

Another said that:

21/5 6/40–42
If you respect your student that filters down (to patient care).

Table 6.41
Caring for students and caring for patients (n=12)

Properties:

1 It's different the way I care for students as compared to how I cared for patients. 3 responses
2 Caring for students and patients is similar because both are about caring for people. 2 responses
3 Because nurse teachers are nurses they act in a caring ways to their students. 2 responses
4 People respond if they are respected by others. 1 response
5 Clinical staff often don't care adequately when no one is caring for them. 1 response
6 Nursing students are well cared for. 1 response
7 I've read that students will role model caring tutor behaviour but I don't know if students would do this consciously. 1 response
8 Students have said to me we learn how to care because we have nurse teachers as role models who care for us. 1 response
9 Nursing students need more care from their teachers than other students because of the problems they encounter in clinical practice. 1 response
10 I have compensated for the loss of my clinical role through transferring caring for my patients to caring for my students. 1 response
11 I would like students to copy how I care for them when they are caring for patients. 1 response
12 I do not care for students to the same extent as I did care for patients. 1 response
13 You may over care for patients but not for students. 1 response
14 Because I care for students my job is made more difficult. 1 response

It may therefore be concluded that the concept of caring for students is important for those interviewed. However, caring for patients is for a number of the interviewees seen as being qualitatively and quantitatively different from caring for students. Nevertheless how pre–registration nursing students are cared for by nurse teachers is seen as important in terms of students replicating this behaviour when delivering patient care.

Summary of the data analysis of the nurse teacher interviews

As described previously, one of the aims of conducting the nurse teacher interviews has been to incorporate a degree of methodological triangulation in the approaches taken to data collection. This has been in order to increase validity of the research findings.

The interview data themes have given insight into how the central question under investigation may be answered. This question being, what are the relationships between how students are taught and how they approach patient care? Thus learning theories, how the role of the nurse teacher is articulated, and nurse teachers' perceptions of caring for patients are thought to be important areas for consideration.

Theme one, for example, addresses the values and perceptions of theories held by the nurse teachers. This theme may be compared with the second data theme of how these learning theories are translated into the delivery of pre–registration nurse education. The final theme relates to nursing value systems of care delivery. Linkage between the themes is therefore attitudes to student–centredness, whether such beliefs are articulated in nurse education, nursing value systems and identification of interconnections between the two value systems. Comparisons of caring for patients with caring for students is therefore a focal issue.

Comparisons between the SAQ survey data and theme one of the interview reveals that negotiation and taking account of individual differences and needs in the teaching and learning process are key concepts attributed to student–centred education in pre–registration nurse training. The importance of self–directed learning and teaching and development of the skills needed for this type of learning generally had consensus. Analysis of the interview data, however, showed that there is no uniform approach to how self–directed learning skills are developed in the individual educational institutions. Some institutions appeared to have made a concerted effort to address the development of such skills through providing study skills modules whereas others had not. Addressing differences in student learning needs and preferences was identified in the factor analysis of the SAQ data as being a unifying concept. However, it was shown in analysis of the interview data that there is little evidence that teaching is tailored to take account of individual learning styles but teachers do generally seem to want to take account of individual learning preferences. Conclusions drawn from the interview data do, however, indicate that it is usually group needs and wishes that are taken account of, rather than those of individual students.

A further way of addressing the needs of individual students is demonstrated to be through use of contract learning. Attitudes to contract learning were shown in SAQ survey as having relatively high disagreement scores. Interview responses, however, showed whilst contract learning was not used in a formalised way in the majority of educational institutions it is used in certain specific circumstances. These circumstances tend to be when individual students are having particular difficulties. Disadvantages to widespread use of contract learning were, however, given, including the resources and motivation needed for its effective use.

The high agreement score with regard to the SAQ statement about use of experiential learning was generally shown as important but its use was more appropriate to teaching certain subject areas. Experiential learning and teaching were seen as referring to classroom–type teaching situations. Also notions of learning through experience or reflective learning was demonstrated in analysis of both sets of data as being of importance. The interview data show that reflection on practice is addressed in a number of institutions through evaluation of clinical practice sessions and students keeping clinical diaries.

The value of problem–solving learning and teaching in both the attitude survey data and interview data was seen to receive general agreement responses. In the interviews it was demonstrated that problem–solving learning and teaching are normally associated with development of skills needed for use of the nursing process. Questions regarding the value of critical thinking skills as a learning outcome of pre–registration nurse education were only addressed in an implied manner in the SAQ survey (and not in the nurse teacher interviews). However, high agreement SAQ responses were obtained.

The statement pertaining to the concept of andragogy in the SAQ survey again had generally agreement scores that teaching children is different from teaching adults. Analysis of interview data confirms these findings and identifies that respect for the social status of adult learners and taking regard of previous learning experiences is of importance. However, whether or not these principles are actually adhered to by nurse educators is thought by some to be debatable. For example, articulation of andragogical principles is shown to be through the type of power relationships that exist between teachers and students. Nurse education in this context was generally described as being teacher–centred. Also taking account of the adult status of nursing students was seen to be questionable by some interviewees as their institutions use attendance registers.

One of the final categories of data analysis in theme one of the interview data addresses the topic of opposing learning theories to that of a student–centred education. Incorporation of behavioural learning theories in nurse education programmes was seen as being desirable by a number of interviewees as it was felt a balanced approach was needed. Behavioural theories were also seen as having particular relevance to skills teaching. Skills acquisition by students was identified by some as an area for concern and one that needs to be addressed in classroom environments.

The second theme concerns the role of the nurse teacher, and begins with identification of how nurse teachers actually use the previously described learning theories in their teaching activities. The results show that a variety of teaching methods are used which fit with both cognitive, andragogical type learning theories and behaviourist theories. How effective teaching methods are seen to be was shown to be related both to the product and process of learning. Both are monitored through quality assurance strategies. However, barriers to teaching and learning prevented a number of those interviewed using their preferred teaching methods and responding to student evaluations. Major barriers included, for example, inadequate classrooms, lack of human and financial resources, and large class sizes. This may be compared to large class size and cohort size which were identified as significant independent variables in the SAQ survey.

Further data categories pertaining to the role of the nurse teacher related to desirable teacher qualities. These were identified as being a facilitator of learning, someone who supports students and allows freedom to learn. This matches a student–centred type teaching model. Personal tutor systems were shown as a way nurse teachers can address needs of individual students against a backdrop of large class sizes and inadequate resources.

Dimensions of the clinical role of the nurse teacher were given in a number of data categories. Generally it was seen as being problematic in terms of teacher resources and institutional commitment. The interviewees generally reported that their clinical teaching role was acting as support person for students when they were undertaking clinical practice. Clinical link systems were seen as maintaining liaison links between the educational institution, students in practice and their mentors. The effectiveness of these links systems was, however, seen as being contentious.

Notions of nurse teachers' clinical credibility were also explored. This was done with regard to how nurse teachers are seen as role models for student nurses when they are learning about nursing. A number of those interviewed felt it was difficult to maintain clinical expertise. Nevertheless, despite these difficulties, the majority thought they were able to do so. However, a minority felt that this was neither possible nor desirable. The idea of nurse teachers acting as role models is seen as being dependent on their clinical credibility. The majority, however, thought that they were not role models for students but would be if students saw them practising in clinical settings.

These findings are seemingly contradictory. Whilst the majority of interviewees saw themselves as being able to maintain their clinical expertise they did not see themselves as role models for their students. This was because students do not see them in clinical practice. Hence it would seem that maintaining clinical expertise was seen as being addressed as a personal issue and largely divorced from the pragmatic issues surrounding clinical teaching and formalised clinical link systems. The lecturer–practitioner role was seen by some as a solution to this dilemma.

Nurse teachers were, however, thought to have some influence on how student nurses learn about nursing. This is seen as being through teachers using examples of their clinical experiences to illustrate their classroom teaching sessions. Finally the most influential people on how students learn about practice are believed to be clinical staff. The students' own peers and patients are also identified as being important.

The final theme in the nurse teacher interview data was patient–centred care. The nursing process was described as being the most desirable way of approaching care delivery. In essence the nursing process was described as being a systematic, problem–solving approach to the delivery of nursing care. There were a number of negative features of the nursing process identified, not least of these being that it was poorly used in clinical areas.

Data analysis showed that conceptual models of nursing were believed to give a formalised philosophical base to how the nursing process is articulated in practice.

However, personal belief systems were found to be of more importance for those interviewed. These personal belief systems identified similar values to humanistic philosophy. For example, central to both was recognition of the individual, their humanness and the rights of the individual. A further data category in this theme identified how the ideal was that patients are involved in decisions regarding their nursing care and this thereby embraces humanistic philosophical tenets. Patient involvement was shown to be variable and dependent on attitudes in the individual clinical areas and of the individual patients.

The final category of the nurse teacher interview data addressed caring for patients and caring for students. It was shown that how students were cared for by the nurse teachers was seen as important in terms of how they learned to care for patients. However, caring for student nurses was seen as different in terms of the quality and quantity of the input from nurse teachers. Clearly of equal importance also was how nurse education programmes were taught. The inter–relationships between caring and teaching dimensions of the nurse teacher role will be a focus in the following chapter pertaining to discussion of the findings of this study.

The following section of this chapter examines the responses of pre–registration student nurses to similar topic areas in both the SAQ survey and the nurse teacher interviews.

Student nurse questionnaire data analysis

As described in the previous chapter, the next area of data collection involved conducting a questionnaire survey of pre–registration student nurses. The survey was directed to exploring attitudes to student–centred learning and teaching through responses obtained to statements given in a questionnaire. A further aim of the student nurse survey was to establish patient–centredness scores as measured using the PMQX measuring tool. A small pilot study was conducted in two educational institutions with a sample of 30 pre–registration student nurses. One student group was undertaking a undergraduate degree programme while the other was of diploma level. From the results of the pilot study amendments were made to the questionnaire, which was then distributed to a sample of 224 pre–registration student nurses from 10 educational establishments in England.

Student nurse questionnaire sample details

The criteria for selecting the student nurse sample were described in chapter 5. However to summarize, the institutions approached with regard to providing access to a potential student nurse sample were selected on the basis of their crude SAQ scores. Institutions who obtained low, medium low, medium, medium high and high scores were selected and also a representative range of institutions which offered either undergraduate degree or diploma level courses.

The biographical details of the student nurse sample conform to the common characteristics identified by Lathean (1987) in a survey of nurses. For example, the majority in the sample are females (n=185 – 84.37%), are aged between 20 years and 29 years (n=127 – 56.70%). Males (n=39 – 17.41%) and mature student or those over 40 years (n=16 – 7.14%) are therefore the least represented in the sample. Those undertaking adult nursing formed the largest group (n=164 –73.21%) in terms of Branch programme options, whilst those undertaking mental handicap nursing (n=14 –6.25%) were the smallest student group. Numbers of students undertaking diploma level course were in the majority (n=157 – 70.09%), compared to those undertaking undergraduate degree courses (n=67 – 29.91%). Biographical details of the total main study sample are given in appendix 6.

Student nurse questionnaire data analysis (student–centred learning and teaching section)

As identified in previous chapters the main method of data analysis with regard to responses to the student–centred learning and teaching section of the questionnaire was content analysis. This analysis had as a central feature a search for commonalities in responses. Similar responses were therefore grouped together into topic areas pertaining to each question posed in the questionnaire. Numerical values were also calculated regarding topic areas identified. Each set of data has been subsequently tabulated, with majority responses featured at the beginning of each table and minority responses at the end.

The following section of data analysis examines responses obtained to each open–ended question about student–centred learning and teaching.

Statement One   The most important features of student–centred learning for me is as follows

The first question in the student nurse questionnaire is what the sample believed to be the most important features of student–centred learning. Table 6.42 gives the responses obtained. It can be seen from the table that teachers' conduct towards students formed the largest group of response. (n=91, 48.92%). The responses identify that the student nurses respondents surveyed see as important being treated as individuals with regard to their learning needs, being treated with respect and as adult, having independence in learning, and negotiation and partnership between students and teachers. Addressing the individual learning needs of individuals and empowerment of learners can therefore be identified as a key subject areas. These areas were also addressed in the SAQ survey where it was identified that there were largely positive responses to the statements pertaining to nurse teachers negotiating with students regarding the teaching and learning methods used. However, individuality in terms of taking account of individual learning preferences and learning style profiles received in the majority mid–range responses. In the nurse teacher interviews students taking responsibility for their own learning was a key area

Table 6.42
The most important features of student–centred learning for me is as follows (n=186)

Subject areas of the content analysis:

1 Teacher conduct towards students. Responses 91 (48.92%)
2 Teaching is appropriate for nursing practice. Responses 41 (22.04%)
3 Desirable teacher attributes. Responses 38 (20.43%)
4 Self–directed learning. Responses 17 (9.14%)
5 Adequate learning resources. Responses 9 (4.84%)
6 Adequate nursing practice experiences. Responses 8 (4.30%)
7 Desirable student attributes. Responses 8 (4.30%)
8 Being in receipt of peer support. Responses 6 (3.22%)
9 Assessment of learning. Responses 5 (2.69%)
10 Use of certain teaching methods. Responses 5 (2.69%)

I don't know what it means/not answered by 38 (20.43%)

in terms of how the nurse teachers interviewed define student–centred learning and teaching. Nevertheless choice and negotiation regarding the learning process and students identifying their own needs were seen as being of major importance.The second major area identified by the student nurse respondents is with regard to being taught adequate and appropriate knowledge as necessary for nursing practice (41 responses 22.04%). This area can be shown to match to the nurse teacher interviews. For example, with regard to teaching and learning methods table 6.26 shows that some nurse teachers interviewed identified students want the straight forward delivery of 'facts'. Of clear importance to the student nurse respondents is the eventual outcome of nurse educational programmes of being equipped with the knowledge and skills necessary for nursing practice.

The third major area identified is desirable teacher attributes (38 responses 20.43%). Supportive teachers and teachers who deliver informative and interesting sessions are seen as being important. There are no direct comparisons possible between these responses and those of the institutional questionnaire. However, comparisons with the nurse teacher data show similar areas of concern. In table 6.28, which is in regard of desirable nurse teacher qualities, features identified by a number of nurse teachers, include that the delivery of information in sessions is enjoyable and humorous (see table 6.26). However, an over–riding theme is that desirable teacher attributes are seen more in terms of being a facilitator of learning as against a deliver of information (see tables 6.11 and 6.12). The nurse teachers interviewed also see support of students as an important part of their role.

Self–directed learning is a further theme identified in responses to this statement (17 responses – 9.14%). Whilst this is examined in more detail by a direct question relating to self–directed learning, it should be noted that self–directed learning as one of the facets of student–centred learning and teaching can be shown to arise as a spontaneous feature of how student–centredness is perceived by the student nurses surveyed.

Other subject areas identified from the student nurse questionnaire data relating to the features of student–centred learning are seen to be of less importance as they all received less than 5% of the responses. Examples of these are adequate learning resources (9 responses – 4.84%) which may be compared to the barriers to preferred methods of teaching (see table 6.28) in the nurse teacher interviews. However, where the nurse teachers identified particular under–resourced areas, the students merely identified adequate resources are necessary. Desirable student attributes form a further small subject area (8 responses – 4.30%) which may be compared to how the nurse teachers interviewed defined student–centred learning (see table 6.11). Whereas the teachers saw student nurses taking responsibility for their own learning as an important part of student–centred learning and teaching, only a relatively small number of student nurses commented on this. Thus it can be inferred as being of less importance to students. Other areas with small numbers of responses attributed to them relate to the importance of peer support (6 responses – 3.22%), assessment criteria (5 responses – 2.69) and teaching methods (5 responses – 2.68%).

Statement Two   Self–directed learning is an important feature of my course

The second statement on the student nurse questionnaire addresses the topic area of self–directed learning and the relative emphasis placed upon it in courses of studies. The responses displayed in table 6.43 demonstrate overall agreement that self–directed learning is an important feature of the respondents' courses (69 responses – 31.65%). This may be compared with the results of the SAQ survey, where overall high agreement scores were obtained regarding self–directed learning (see table 6.1).

Comparisons of student nurses' responses with those of nurse teachers (see table 6.15) show similar areas of agreement. However, teachers placed relatively more importance on students having some basic knowledge of a subject area as a prerequisite for self–directed learning activities. Whilst some of the student nurses surveyed did see this as important, these comments formed the smallest percentage of responses (4 responses – 1.83%).

There is also agreement between the two groups in terms of students needing support and guidance from teachers. It can be identified from both sets of data that this support and guidance is not always adequate. Control of personal learning was seen also as important to the student respondents (28 responses – 12.84%), which links with the nurse teacher comments that self–directed learning makes students more autonomous in their learning. However, further comparisons may be also made with table 6.22 regarding power relationships. Here it is identified by nurse teacher interviewees that power still rests with the teacher and the institution.

It is seen in a number of the nurse teacher responses that students' abilities to undertake self–directed learning activities may be under–estimated when compared with the majority of comments made by the student nurses, whilst a number of student nurse respondents identify that self–motivation is essential for successful self–directed learning (16 responses – 7.34%). A number also identified that they lacked such motivation and that undertaking self–directed learning is difficult for a variety of reasons (14 responses – 6.42%). From these last points it can inferred that the student nurses see themselves has being capable of coping with self directed learning but for some there is a lack of motivation or they are prevented from undertaking self–directed for other reasons. Similar issues regarding self–motivation are, however, identified by one nurse teacher interviewed (see table 6.13).

Self–directed learning as associated with personal development (24 responses – 11.01%) and acquiring knowledge (23 responses –10.55%) is seen as relatively important by student nurse respondents. However, these areas do not have any explicit comparisons in the nurse teacher interview data. Also identified in the student nurse survey is the fact that generally more time needs to be allocated for self–directed learning (7 responses – 3.21%) and further study of topics introduced in lectures is needed (11 responses – 5.05%).

Categories which represent less than 5% of the total responses relate to the need for increased self–directed learning as the course progresses (5 responses –2.29%), resources need to be adequate (4 responses – 1.83%), and in order successfully to complete the course self directed learning is vital (4 responses – 1.83%). The last topic, as with some previously discussed demonstrates the mportance to the student nurses of the end product of their learning and its assessment. This may be compared with the nurse teachers concerns and their greater emphasis on the process of teaching.

Table 6.43

Self–directed learning (SDL) is an important feature of my course (n=218)

Subject areas of the content analysis:

1 Positive. Responses 69 (31.65%)
2 Support, guidance and feedback from teachers is important but is not always adequate. Responses 32 (14.68%)
3 SDL allows me control over my own learning. Responses 28 (12.84%)
4 SDL helps personal development and gives the opportunity to concentrate on personal weaknesses. Responses 24 (11.01%)
5 SDL is important as it allows me to learn more. Responses 23 (10.55%)
6 Self–motivation is important for SDL. Responses 16 (7.34%) 7
7 Negative. Responses 16 (7.34%)
8 Undertaking SDL is sometimes difficult. Responses 14 (6.42%)
9 SDL is important as private study is needed after lectures. Responses 11 (5.05%)
10 SDL gives me motivation to learn and increases my learning capacity. Responses 10 (4.59%)
11 SDL is important with regard to assessments. Responses 9 (4.13%)
12 More SDL time needs to be allocated. Responses 7 (3.21%)
13 Allocation of SDL time is sometimes abused by teachers. Responses 6 (2.75%)
14 Teachers give support and guidance with regard to SDL activites. Responses 6 (2.75%)
15 SDL is more important at different stages of the course. Responses 5 (2.29%)
16 SDL is a prerequisite for successful completion of the course. Responses 4 (1.83%)

Table 6.43 cont:

Subject areas of the content analysis: cont

17 The resources available are not always adequate for SDL. Responses 4 (1.83%)

18 Adequate knowledge of the subject area is a prerequisite of SDL. Responses 4 (1.83%)

Unanswered by 6 (2.75%) respondents

Statement Three I have been taught self–directed learning skills on my course

Table 6.43 gives the student nurse responses to whether self–directed learning skills are taught on their courses. It can be seen that negative responses were obtained from just over 40% (86 responses) of the sample with some identifying more help and guidance is needed (11 responses – 5.24%). Affirmative responses were less than 30% (59 responses). These responses may be compared with table 6.1 pertaining to the SAQ survey, where there are generally high agreement scores regarding the statement that self–directed learning skills are taught in the institution. Also in the nurse teacher data there is general agreement that self–directed learning skills are taught in the institution (see table 6.13). For example, study skills are identified by the nurse teachers as being incorporated into the majority of programmes they are involved with.

Similarly some of the smaller response categories of the student nurse responses do identify some study skills been taught (54 responses – 24.71%), nurse teachers as helping students develop these skills (8 responses – 3.80%) and a number of ways study skills–type topics (6 responses –2.86%) have been introduced in their course.

However, generally it can be shown from the student nurse data that self–directed learning skills were seen as being an under–addressed area. For example, a number of the student nurse respondents identify that, whilst they have been taught these skills, further teaching and support is needed (21 responses – 10.00%). Comments also relate to that students had developed these skills themselves (17 responses – 8.09%). However, a number also stated that they had developed these skills in educational courses they had undertaken previously (15 responses – 7.14%). Also identified was that it may be questionable if the requisite skills can be taught at all because they were perceived as being a natural ability (5 responses – 2.38%).

Table 6.44

I have been taught self–directed learning skills on my course (n=210)

Subject areas of the content analysis:

1 Negative. Responses 86 (40.95%)

2 Affirmative. Responses 59 (28.09%)

3 Certain subject areas taught and associated with developing SDL skills. Responses 54 (25.71%).

4 SDL skills are taught but not effectively/with no reinforcement. Responses 21 (10.00%)

5 SDL skills have been self taught. Responses 17 (8.09%)

Table 6.44 cont:

Subject areas of the content analysis: cont

6 Students already had these skills or are capable of managing their own learning. Responses 15 (7.14%)
7 SDL activities need teacher support, guidance and follow–up. Responses 11 (5.24%)
8 SDL skills are dependent on self–motivation/commonsense. Responses 8 (3.80%)
9 Certain teachers have helped students developed their SDL skills. Responses 8 (3.80%)
10 Certain teaching methods used by teachers help the development of SDL skills. Responses 6 (2.86%)
11 SDL skills cannot be taught as they need to be developed by individuals. Responses 5 (2.38%)

Unanswered by 14 (6.66%) repondents

Statement Four Active learning is an important feature of my course

Table 6.45 gives the student nurse responses to if active learning is an important feature of their educational programme. It can be shown generally that positive responses predominate (111 responses – 52.85%). These responses may be compared with the institutional attitude survey (see table 6.1) where there is general overall agreement to the statement that student–centred learning and teaching means active learning.

Comparisons with the nurse teacher interviews may be made through analysis of the category pertaining to experiential learning (see table 6.18). It can be demonstrated in the nurse teacher interviews that active learning was for the majority seen in the context of classroom teaching and learning activities. However, whilst the largest category of responses from the student nurses refer to active learning in a classroom, a substantial percentage of responses do refer to active learning in clinical practice (40 responses – 19.05%). Furthermore in other categories the student nurses reported a need for more clinical practice and practical skills training (26 responses – 12.38%). Also identified was the importance of integrating theory and practice (15 responses – 7.14%). These points are not duplicated in the nurse teacher interview data.

There is also an emphasis in the student nurse data on how active learning methods develop personal attributes and, as discussed in previously analysed student nurse data, how active learning increases knowledge of subject areas (37 responses – 17.61%). However, in the nurse teacher data the emphasis is experience of how patients may possibly feel rather than acquiring knowledge and learning 'facts' as in the student nurse data.

Issues which accrued small percentages of comments concerned active learning giving variety to learning and teaching methods (9 responses – 4.28%), and the need for all students to participate in active learning activities (9 responses – 4.28%). For example, equal participation in group–work was cited by a number of the respondents. Negative comments were also made in response to the statement. For example, active learning methods are disliked by some students (7 responses – 3.33%) and that these methods are under–utilised in their course programme (7 responses – 3.33%). As with responses to previous questions a small proportion of students report that more support from teachers is needed (6 responses –2.86%).

Table 6.45

Active learning is an important feature of my course (n=210)

Subject areas of the content analysis:

1 Positive. Responses 111 (52.85%)
2 AL is related to clinical nursing experience. Responses 40 (19.05%)
3 AL helps develop personal attributes/assists learning. Responses 37 (17.61%)
4 More clinical practice/clinical teaching is needed on my course. Responses 26 (12.38%)
5 AL helps me relate theory to practice. Responses 15 (7.14%)
6 AL helps maintain interest in the subject being taught and gives variety. Responses 9 (4.28%)
7 Individual participation in AL teaching is important. Responses 9 (4.28%)
8 AL is important but there is not enough use of it on my course. Responses 7 (3.33%)
9 AL is not always an effective teaching method. Responses 7 (3.33%)
10 AL is part of self–directed learning. Responses 7 (3.33%)
11 More guidance and support is needed from teachers in regard to AL. Responses 6 (2.86%)
12 More effective co-ordination of theory and practice is needed. Responses 3 (1.43%)
13 AL is not an important feature of my course. Responses 8 (3.81%)

Unanswered by 14 (6.66%) respondents

Statement Five Problem–solving skills are taught on my course

Responses regarding problem–solving skills are displayed in table 6.46. As shown in analysis of data pertaining to previous questions there is a relatively high response rate (204 responses – 91.07%). However, this question received the lowest number of responses. Generally comments were of a negative nature (96 responses – 47.05%) or that more problem–solving skills needed to be taught (23 responses – 11.27%). This may be compared with the SAQ survey where there was unequivocal agreement with the statement that student–centred teaching and learning involve problem–solving activities. There were similar responses to the SAQ survey, indicating that critical thinking skills are a valued educational outcome of pre–registration nurse education programmes.

Comparisons with the nurse teacher interview data give similar disparities between responses of students and those of nurse teachers. The nurse teachers interviewed generally perceived that problem–solving skills were taught in their pre–registration programmes (see table 6.20). This may be further contrasted to the generally negative nature of the student nurse responses.

Both the nurse teacher and student nurse groups identified problem–solving skills as being inter–related to teaching and learning about use of the nursing process and nursing theory teaching (16 responses – 7.84%). However, a small number of student nurse responses do refer to teaching and learning of problem–solving as being left to be taught whilst students are in clinical practice (10 responses – 4.90%). As with previously analysed areas of the student nurse data, there are conflicting views regarding the support and guidance that nurse teachers give to students (5 responses – 2.45%).

It is also identified in the student nurse data that problem–solving skills are perceived as being taught with regards to other subject areas (20 responses – 9.80%). These subject areas included, for example, moral and ethical reasoning, management studies and study skills programmes. Certain teaching and learning strategies are also seen as assisting students to develop their problem–solving skills (16 responses – 7.84%). However, a case–study approach, whilst thought by some to be generally a good teaching strategy, was seen by others as unsatisfactory (3 responses – 1.47%).

Table 6.46

Problem–solving skills are taught on my course (n=204)

Subject areas of the content analysis:

1 Negative Replies - Responses 96 (47.05%)
2 Positive Replies - Responses 46 (22.55%)
3 More teaching/more effective teaching is needed with regard to PPS. Responses 23 (11.27%)
4 PPS are taught in certain modules. Responses 20 (9.80%)
5 PPS are taught in nursing studies modules. Responses 16 (7.84%)
6 PPS are developed through use of certain teaching methods. Responses 16 (7.84%)
7 PPS are taught/will be taught in clinical practice. Responses 10 (4.90%)
8 Some teachers help students develop PPS. Responses 6 (2.94%)
9 Teachers do not give enough guidance in respect of the development of students' PPS. Responses 5 (2.45%)
10 The case studies used for problem–solving exercises are inadequate/under–used. Responses 3 (1.47%)
11 PPS cannot be taught as they are about common sense. Responses 3 (1.47%)

Unanswered by 16 (7.84%) respondents

Statement Six I prefer the following teaching/learning methods

Table 6.47 gives the preferred teaching methods of the student nurses in the sample. There are no direct comparisons with this data and the SAQ survey data. However, questions were asked in the SAQ survey regarding taking account of student nurses preferred teaching and learning methods and individual learning styles (see table 6.1).

Responses to both these statements revealed no clear consensus on whether or not regard is taken of student nurses' learning styles or learning preferences. Other statements in the SAQ survey also indirectly relate to this question. For example, the statement pertaining to nurse teachers negotiating with students regarding teaching and learning methods received slightly more positive than negative responses (see table 6.1). Similarly, the statement about contract learning received no clear pattern of negative or positive responses (see table 6.1).

In the nurse teacher data, as discussed previously, it was shown that the teachers defined student–centred learning and teaching in terms of permitting choice and negotiation (see table 6.11). This theme is also a focus of table 6.15, where it was shown that the majority of the nurse teachers see taking account of students' learning preferences as important. However, it was also demonstrated in analysis of the nurse teacher interview data that student nurses' individual needs cannot often be a main focus and teaching is usually directed towards catering for group needs (see table 6.16).

Direct comparisons with the nurse teacher data and the responses obtained from the student nurse questionnaire can be shown through examination of table 6.26 as compared to table 6.47. It is shown that there is a similar inter–mix of responses between both sets of data. For example, the student nurse data show lecture–type teaching and learning activities as accruing the majority of responses (74 responses – 33.94%) which is similar to responses of the nurse teachers. However, a salient feature of the remainder of the preferred methods of teaching and learning the student nurses identify are that they are those usually associated with active student–participative learning activities.

It would, however, seem generally from the variety of responses in the student nurse data that there is no one method that meets all the individual student nurse preferences. Indeed it was noted that a large number replies identified preferences for a number of differing methods. These included, for example, a combination of lectures, self–directed learning activities, group–work strategies, seminars and tutorials. This, coupled with the section of the student nurse data related to the use of teaching aids (39 responses – 17.89%) leads to conclusions that use of a variety of teaching methods which are also visually stimulating is important.

It is also identified in the student data is that clinical practice is an important learning activity (31 responses –14.22%). Both students and teachers see skills training as important (see table 6.26 for the nurse teacher data), but a larger number of student nurse responses refer to learning in practice. Also it is demonstrated by a number of student nurse responses that there is a perceived need for more clinical practice in their courses.

Small subject areas are also identified in the student nurse data which may be compared with both the SAQ data and the nurse teacher data. For example, a relatively small number of student nurse respondents identify that they enjoy reflection on practice sessions (4 responses – 1.83%). This may be compared to high agreement responses in the SAQ survey (see table 6.1) and the nurse teacher interview data (see table 6.19). It is concluded, therefore in view of the small number of student responses that reflection on practice as a preferred teaching and learning method is of less importance to the student nurses than to nurse teachers.

Finally it should be noted that there is no reference made by the student nurse respondents to the use of learning contracts. This may be compared with the ambivalent responses recorded in the results of the SAQ survey. Furthermore the nurse teacher data also identifies problems with the use of learning contracts on a large scale basis, with a general consensus being that they are more suitable for use with individuals who have special learning needs.

Table 6.47

I prefer the following teaching/learning methods (n=218)

Content analysis subject areas:

1 Lectures. Responses 74 (33.94%)
2 Group work. Responses 45 (20.64%)
3 Comments with regard to the use of certain teaching aids. Response 39 (17.89%)
4 Self–directed learning/private study. Responses 35 (16.05%)
5 Group discussions/debates. Responses 34 (15.59%)
6 Seminars. Responses 33 (15.13%)
7 Practical experience. Responses 31 (14.22%)
8 Lectures with student participation. Responses 27 (12.38%)
9 Active learning methods. Responses 25 (11.46%)
10 Tutorials/small group teaching/individual teaching. Responses 23 (10.55%)
11 Lectures followed by other learning activities. Responses 22 (10.09%)
12 Certain teaching methods that are disliked. Responses 22 (10.09%)
13 Practical skills training. Responses 14 (6.42%)
14 A variety of methods/interesting teaching/teaching that is fun. Responses 13 (5.96%)
15 Student participation/teaching interacting. Responses 13 (5.96%)
16 Being able to relate theory to practice. Responses 7 (3.21%)
17 Assignments/examinations/tests. Responses 5 (2.29%)
18 Reflective sessions. Responses 4 (1.83%)

Unanswered by 6 respondents (2.75%)

Statement Seven I have been treated as an adult by the majority of people I have come in contact with on my course so far

Table 6.48 displays responses of the student nurses regarding if they have been treated is an adult by the majority of people they have come into contact with on their course. This data may be compared with the SAQ survey with regard to the statement pertaining to the principles of teaching adults being different from those of teaching children. Responses to the SAQ survey give overall patterns of positive responses thereby, giving some evidence of beliefs in andragogical tenets. The nurse teacher data gives a similar category of responses (see table 6.21). However, nurse teacher data shows that whilst andragogy as a theory is generally endorsed, it is seen as being debatable by some of those interviewed whether or not it is actually practised.

Student nurse responses regarding whether they are treated as adults on their courses gives the largest positive result of any of the statements so far. It is shown that 69.20% (155 responses) of the respondents give affirmative responses to this question which, is therefore contradictory to the nurse teacher data. However, a small percentage of the student nurse responses are negative in nature regarding nurse teacher/institutional attitudes towards students (35 responses – 15.83%). It can be also shown that a relatively high number of student nurses also think staff in clinical areas accord student nurses adult status (24 responses – 10.85%), whilst previous responses have shown that some student nurses want more clinical practice, it is shown in this section that their treatment on clinical placement may sometimes be suspect.

Other themes of the student nurses' responses regarding their adult status identify that attitudes towards them may vary according to their stage of training (12 responses – 5.43%). For example, a number of responses to refer to attitudes to students at the beginning of their course and especially when undertaking a Common Foundation Programme as being markedly different from when they have progressed further on in their training and entered Branch programmes.

Also shown in the student nurse data is the fact that attitudes to some younger members of student groups are different from attitudes towards the mature members of the group (12 responses – 5.43%). However, a number of the younger respondents identify that it is not necessarily nurse teachers' attitudes towards them which are not in keeping with andragogical tenets: some replies identify that mature students' treatment of younger students could sometimes be the subject of criticism.

Table 6.48

I have been treated as an adult by the majority of people I have come into contact with on my course so far (n=221)

Content analysis subject areas:

1 Positive Replies. Responses 155 (69.20%)
2 Negative Replies. Responses 35 (15.83%)
3 Staff in the clinical areas do not treat students as adults. Responses 24 (10.85%)
4 Was not treated as an adult at the beginning of the course. Responses 19 (8.59%)
5 Because I am a younger student I am not treated as an adult. Responses 12 (5.43%)
6 The teachers/institution respects our adult status. Responses 11 (4.97%)
7 The use of registers undermines our adult status. Responses 10 (4.52%)
8 Some teaching methods used are not in keeping with respecting our adult status. Responses 5 (2.26%)
9 Staff in the clinical areas treat students as adults. Responses 5 (2.26%)
10 My peers treat me as an adult. Responses 3 (1.35%)
11 As a mature student I expect to be treated as an adult. Responses 2 (0.90%)

Unanswered by 3 (1.35%) respondents

Smaller sections of the data in table 6.48 can be compared with issues established from the nurse teacher data. For example, a number of the student nurses saw use of class registers as undermining their adult status (10 responses – 4.52%). Table 6.23 which pertains to the nurse teacher interview data, shows that a relatively small number of those interviewed commented that class registers were used in their institution. One teacher interviewee also saw this in terms of negating the adult status of student nurses.

Further small sections of data in table 6.48 refer to use of some teaching methods as not being appropriate with adult learners (5 responses – 2.26%). For example, experiential teaching and learning methods appeared to be disliked by a small number of students. Other sections of data give contradictory evidence to previously discussed topics regarding positive attitudes of clinical staff (5 responses – 2.60%) and the students' peer towards the respondents (3 responses –1.35%).

Statement Eight The most effective way I have learnt about nursing has been as follows

Table 6.49 gives the student nurse responses to the question of what is perceived as the most effective way to learn about nursing. There are no directly comparable questions in the SAQ survey or in the nurse teacher interviews.

Responses obtained from the student nurses regarding learning about nursing show a large majority relating to learning about clinical nursing practice (130 responses – 59.09%). Effective clinical placements are shown to be of key importance to the student nurse respondents. Other smaller categories of data also relate to the importance of clinical practice to the students surveyed (22 responses – 10.00%). Contact with nurses is identified important, as is contact with patients (10 responses – 4.54%). Experiences in the past of nursing practice were also seen by some as having a significant influence (11 responses – 5.00%). As seen in previous sections of the data some of the student nurses also thought there should be more clinical practice in their course (14 responses – 6.35%).

Table 6.49

The most effective way I have learnt about nursing is as follows (n=220)

Subject areas of the content analysis:

1 Practical nursing experience. Responses 130 (59.09%)
2 Through a combination of theory and practice. Responses 36 (16.36%)
3 Through self–directed study activities. Responses 30 (13.64%)
4 Through practical skills training. Responses 23 (10.45%)
5 Through contact with nurses. Responses 22 (10.00%)
6 Through being exposed to certain teaching methods. Responses 20 (9.90%)
7 More nursing practice needs to be included and more relevant/less theory. Responses 14 (6.36%)
8 From previous experiences of nursing. Responses 11 (5.00%)

Table 6.49 cont:

Subject areas of the content analysis: cont

9 By sharing nursing experiences. Responses 11 (5.00%)
10 Through the influence of nurse teachers. Responses 10 (4.54%)
11 Through contact with patients/clients. Responses 10 (4.54%)
12 From by fellow students. Responses 8 (3.63%)
13 By learning about nursing theory. Responses 8 (3.63%
14 Through work done for assignments. Responses 7 (3.18%)
15 Through learning about theoretical disciplines applies to nursing. Responses 5 (2.27%)
16 Through observing poor/inadequate nursing practice. Responses 2 (0.91%)
Unanswered by 4 (1.82%) respondents

A very small number of respondents also thought they had learnt from observing poor or inadequate nursing practice (2 responses – 0.91%).

Whilst some of the student nurses thought there should be less or more relevant nursing theory, it was identified by a larger numbers that both the theory taught and nursing practice were of equal importance (36 responses – 16.36%). An inter–mix of teaching methods such as, for example, self–directed learning activities (30 responses – 13.64%), lectures, group work activities, seminars and tutorials (20 responses – 9.90%) are again seen as being effective when learning about nursing.

Some student nurse respondents also identify practical skills training as being important (23 responses – 10.45%). This compares to a similar category of data established from the nurse teacher interviews (see table 6.25). The nurse teachers gave similar responses to the student nurses in that both groups think that practical skills training is an area of concern and sometimes more teaching of practical skills is needed.

Sharing nursing experiences with others is also seen as being beneficial to the student nurses (11 responses – 5.00%). However, there is no explicit evidence that this is related to reflection on practice sessions, as discussed previously. Finally nurse teachers are seen by a number of respondents as having an important influence, especially 'good' teachers who are up–to–date with clinical practice and appropriately relate the theory they are teaching to nursing practice. Comparisons with nurse teachers' perceptions of their influence on students learning about nursing are analysed in depth in the following section.

Statement Nine The most influential people for me learning about nursing have as follows

Table 6.50 gives the student nurse responses to which people are seen as being influential when the student nurses are learning about nursing. There are no comparable questions in the SAQ survey. However, a number of categories in the nurse teacher data interrelate with this question.

The most frequently cited influential group are nurse teachers (131 responses – 62.38%). Of direct comparison to these responses are the data displayed in table 6.35, where the nurse teachers generally did not see themselves as important role models for student nurses because students did not see them practising in clinical settings. The clinical role of the nurse teacher is given in table 6.31. In this table a number of nurse teachers identify that they make clinical practice visits to students but the majority do not undertake a clinical teaching role. In table 6.32 which pertains to clinical link systems such systems are generally identified as needing improvement. Similarly table 6.33 demonstrates that maintaining clinical credibility is difficult, with some nurse teachers commenting that they do nursing agency work in order to maintain their clinical competence. The most influential people regarding how student nurse learn about nursing in the nurse teachers' perceptions are shown in table 6.35. Again it is seen that clinical staff are thought to have the most influence. It may therefore be generally concluded that the nurse teachers interviewed, in comparison to the student nurse responses, underestimated the influence they have on student nurses in terms of learning about nursing.

Other sections of data concerning student responses do, however, identify the importance of clinical staff's role (117 responses – 55.71%) and particularly the students' ward mentors (67 responses – 31.90%). Patients and other health care professionals (8 responses – 3.81%) are also seen as being a significant influence. So whilst the large group of student nurse comments related to nurse teachers', a large proportion of comments do also interrelate with learning in clinical practice.

The student nurse data also identify other socialising influences as being friends and relatives (11 responses – 5.24%) and the students' own peers (45 responses – 21.42%). A small percentage of responses also make negative comments about nurse teachers' roles (8 responses – 3.81%). As already discussed some also see previous nursing experiences as being influential (3 responses – 1.42%) and themselves and their personal experiences as also being important (7 responses – 3.33%).

Table 6.50

The most influential people for me learning about nursing have been as follows (n=210)

Subject areas of the content analysis:

1 Nurse teachers. Responses 131 (62.38%)
2 Clinical staff. Responses 117 (55.71%)
3 Mentors. Responses 67 (31.90%)
4 Other students. Responses 45 (21.42%)
5 Patients. Responses 21 (10.00%)
6 Friends and relatives. Responses 11 (5.24%)
7 Negative comments about nurse teachers. Responses 8 (3.81%)
8 Other health care professionals. Responses 8 (3.81%)
9 Myself and my personal experiences. Responses 7 (3.33)
10 Previous experiences. Responses 3 (1.42%)
11 Other influences mentioned.
Librarians 1 response
TV programmes such as Casualty 1 response
Research findings 1 response

Table 6.50 cont:

Subject areas of the content analysis: cont

- Text books such as Roper et al 1 response
- Group work 1 response
- God 1 response

Not answered by 14 (6.67%) respondents

It may be concluded from this section that there is a multiplicity of people who are seen to exert influence on student nurses' learning about nursing. Indeed, as with responses to other questions, the responses obtained to this question frequently give a number of important influences rather than citing one over–riding influence.

Statement Ten I feel valued as an individual by the majority of people I have come into contact with whilst on my course

The final section of data analysis regarding the student nurses surveyed deals with whether they feel valued as individuals by the majority of people they have come into contact with whilst on their course. There are no comparable questions in the SAQ survey. However, a number of the nurse teacher interview data categories interrelate to this topic.

Generally it can be seen that the student nurses surveyed do feel valued as individuals (121 responses – 57.07%). A small number also identify that being cared for as students is important in terms of learning how to care for patients. This may be compared with table 6.41, where it is shown that the majority of nurse teachers interviewed thought that caring for students was important although for some it was different in terms of the quality and quantity of care given to patients. A number of interviewees also identify the importance of a role modelling effect. For example, teachers' caring attitudes towards students are replicated by the students when they are caring for patients. Positive comments made by the student nurses (20 responses – 9.43%) also specifically identify nurse teachers and personal tutors as valuing students' individuality. These responses can be compared with table 6.30 which shows generally that the nurse teachers think that personal tutor systems permit a humanistic, personal response to individual students' needs.

A substantial percentage of negative comments (39 responses – 18.39%) were, however, made by the student nurse respondents regarding nurse teacher attitudes. A number identified that often teachers do not know them individually by name. These responses may be compared to table 6.12 regarding the nurse teacher interviews, where similar areas of concern were expressed. Generally the nurse teachers thought, because of large number of students they come into contact with, that maintaining an individual approach is often difficult. Large group numbers are also identified in table 6.28 pertaining to barriers to the use of preferred teaching and learning methods. In addition analysis of the SAQ survey data shows that there are significantly differing responses in terms of taking account of individual learning styles and institutions with medium high cohort sizes.

Smaller categories of the student nurse responses to being valued as an individual give diverse evidence regarding similar topic areas. For example, a relatively large number of responses (27 responses – 12.73%) pertain to negative comments regarding students' experiences in clinical practice. This may be compared to previous areas of discussion where, although students identify the need for more clinical practice, attitudes to them whilst undertaking practical placements may be dubious. However, smaller numbers of positive responses can be shown with regard to clinical practice (19 responses – 8.96%). Similarly there are a number of positive comments regarding students' peer groups (12 responses – 5.66%) which are offset by to a smaller number of negative comments (5 responses – 2.36%). Finally a small number of student nurse responses also relate to the fact that the type of course they are doing sometimes has a bearing on being treated as an individual (10 responses – 4.72%).

Table 6.51
I feel valued as an individual by the majority of people I have come into contact with whilst on my course (n=212)

Subject areas of the content analysis:

1 Positive Replies. Responses 121 (57.07%)
2 Negative comments with regard to teachers/institution. Responses 39 (18.39%)
3 Negative comments with regards of clinical placements. Responses 27 (12.73%)
4 Positive responses with regard to teachers/institution. Responses 20 (9.43%)
5 Positive comments with regard to placements. Responses 19 (8.96%)
6 General negative comments. Responses 16 (7.55%)
7 Positive comments in respect of students' peers. Responses 12 (5.66%)
8 There are too many students on my course for me to be valued as an individual. Responses 11 (5.19%)
9 Sometimes there are negative attitudes because I am a student/because of the type of course I am doing. Responses 10 (4.72%)
10 Negative comments about students' own peers. Responses 5 (2.36%)

Unanswered by 12 (5.66%) respondents

Summary of the findings of the student nurse questionnaire data (student–centred learning and teaching section)

As described earlier, one of the aims of the research methods used in this study is to incorporate a degree of methodological triangulation. Therefore where appropriate the findings obtained from the first part of the student nurse questionnaire have been compared with the findings both of the SAQ survey and the nurse teacher interviews. Generally it has been shown there are some consensus findings between the three sets of data. However there is also conflicting evidence pertaining to discrete areas of the data.

Definitions of student–centred learning are the first area addressed with regard to the student nurse responses. The student nurse responses broadly compared with both the SAQ survey findings and the nurse teacher interview data. For example, factor analysis of the SAQ survey data identifies that taking account of individual differences is a major concept. Similarly, it can be identified in analysis of the student nurse data that major features are being treated as an individual and an adult. Also of major importance to the student nurses was being in receipt of effective and appropriate teaching. However, although generally the student nurse questionnaire response rate is high, it should be noted that just over 20% of the student nurse respondents either failed to answer this question or said they were unable to define what student–centred learning meant for them. Emphasis in the nurse teacher responses regarding definitions of student–centred learning and teaching is, however, slightly different. The nurse teacher responses regarding this topic area relate to permitting choice and negotiation in the learning process and student nurses taking responsibility for their own learning.

Questions posed in the student nurse survey regarding self–directed learning and teaching also accrued similar responses to the other three sets of data. All agree that this is an important feature of student–centred learning and an important part the courses of studies the student nurses are undertaking. The student nurses, however, emphasise support and guidance from teachers as essential. The nurse teachers generally appear to underestimate student nurses' abilities to undertake self–directed learning activities as compared with the student nurses.

Responses to the student nurse questionnaire regarding whether or not self–directed learning skills are taught give conflicting evidence when compared with the responses to the SAQ survey and the nurse teacher data. The students are shown generally to feel that such skills are not taught on their courses, whereas both the SAQ survey data and the nurse teacher data demonstrate that it is believed self–directed learning skills are taught in pre–registration nurse education courses.

The question about active learning in the student nurse questionnaire received generally positive responses. These are comparable to the responses received from both the SAQ survey and the nurse teacher interviews. However, the student nurses place an emphasis on active learning with regard to clinical experience, whereas the nurse teachers interpreted active learning as relating to classroom activities.

Conflicting evidence is shown in comparison of the sets of data concerning the question of problem–solving skills. The data from SAQ survey show that it is believed that problem–solving skills are part of student–centred learning and teaching and therefore by implication are taught on pre–registration nurse education programmes. Similarly the nurse teacher data give positive responses and identify problem–solving skills as commonly being taught with regard to use of the nursing process. Whilst generally the student nurse response rate was smaller than those obtained for other questions, negative responses predominate.

The SAQ survey data regarding taking account of individual learning preferences and learning styles gives no clear pattern of responses. Similarly the nurse teacher data gives negative and unclear responses regarding taking account of individual learning styles. However, the data indicate that account is usually taken by the interviewees of group learning and teaching preferences as against individual student nurse learning and teaching preferences. Both the nurse teachers and students data demonstrate that an inter–mix of teaching and learning methods are preferred.

Interesting, appropriate and visually stimulating teaching is identified as important to the student nurses and nurse teachers. There is, therefore, no evidence that teaching and learning methods aligned with a particular theory of learning are utilised by the nurse teachers. Neither does use of a single teaching and learning method appear to be appropriate in terms of the student nurses' preferences.

Convergent responses were obtained in response to questions about andragogy in the SAQ survey and the student nurse responses. Generally both sets of data demonstrate positive responses. The nurse teacher data, whilst being in agreement with the appropriateness of andragogical principles, raised doubts as to whether or not these principles are actually applied in pre-registration nurse education programmes.

Comparisons regarding the data obtained from the nurse teacher interviews and the student nurse survey also give differing responses in terms of people who are influential in how students learn about nursing. Whilst a substantial number of student nurses' responses relate to clinical staff and clinical experiences overall the highest group of positive comments referred to nurse teachers' influence. However, generally the student nurse data features a multiplicity of influential people. In the nurse teacher data, that clinical staff are seen to have the most over-riding influence. The teachers therefore underestimate the importance of their influence on student nurses.

The final question of the student nurse questionnaire pertained to feeling valued as an individual. Whilst the majority of student nurses do feel valued, other substantial areas of data give conflicting evidence. Comparisons with the nurse teacher data show generally that it is felt that student nurses are cared for but this is different from the quality and quantity of care they would give to patients. Both groups do agree that factors such as large student groups, and therefore failure of teachers to know students names', influence feelings of being valued as an individual.

Individuality as one of the previously identified key values of nursing practice is the subject area of the following section, where the student nurses' responses to the PMQX are examined.

Student nurse questionnaire data analysis (PMQX section)

It was shown in the nurse teacher interviews that the nursing process was viewed as a systematic framework for nursing care (see table 6.36) which is often inappropriately used in clinical nursing practice (see table 6.37). Nursing value systems (see table 6.39) were, however, seen in a similar light to features of student-centred learning and teaching as both should address the needs of the individual. Other unifying features of both value systems are those of choice and negotiation in the learning process, which may be compared with patient involvement in decisions regarding their nursing care (see table 6.40). An important feature for student nurses when learning about patient care is, therefore, learning appropriate patient-centred behaviour. The aim of the PMQX as described in the previous chapter is to measure patient-centredness in terms of the responses made to a series of patient care vignettes.

Student nurse questionnaire PMQX section sample details

The student nurse sample for the PMQX section of the questionnaire is the same as that for the previous section of data analysis. However, appendix 6 displays that generally the response rate to the PMQX was lower than to the student-centred learning and teaching section. Whilst there was an overall response rate of 74.17%, the response rate to the PMQX section was 63.58%. As previously described, the overall response rate is deceptive as no students in the main study actually refused to participate. However in the PMQX section there were a number of spoilt and incomplete responses which give rise to the lower response rate.

There are, however, similar biographical features in the PMQX sample of the student nurse questionnaire albeit in differing proportions. Females aged between 20 years and 29 years, those undertaking adult branch studies and those studying at diploma level predomiante, whereas males, those over 40 years, those undertaking mental handicap branch studies and those undertaking degree level programmes are the least represented in the sample.

Statistical analysis of the PMQX data - frequencies, means, medians, and standard deviations

As described in the previous chapter, after data coding the data was analysed using SPSSX. It was also stated that the PMQX instrument is designed to be a global measurement of patient-centredness. Therefore responses to the total questionnaire rather than responses to individual case scenarios are considered.

Table 6.52 gives the frequencies, percentage frequencies, mean, median and standard deviation of the student nurse total PMQX scores. It is shown that the responses are generally distributed normally. However there is a negative skew around the median of 39. These results may be compared to those reported by the author of the PMQX instrument.

Rolfe (1993b) reports a remarkably similar distribution of the scores in a sample of 94 first year Project 2000 diploma students. Rolfe's sample gave scores ranging from a minimum of 25 to a maximum of 47, the mean being 37.775 and the standard deviation 4.413. The results of the present study give a slightly higher mean and standard deviation, which indicates slightly higher average scores and less variability in the range of scores. Nevertheless there is a high degree of comparability between the two sets of data.

Table 6.52
Frequencies, percentage frequencies, mean, median and standard deviation of responses to the PMQX

Values	Frequency	Frequency %
26	1	.5
27	2	.9
30	3	1.4
31	4	1.8
32	3	1.4
33	6	2.8
34	10	4.6
35	10	4.6
36	11	5.0
37	13	6.0
38	20	9.2
39	28	12.8
40		
41	29	13.3
42	16	7.3
43	8	3.7
44	14	6.4
45	7	3.2
46	4	1.8
47	1	.5
Mean 38.96	Median 39.00	SD = 3.83

Rolfe (1993b) gives the significance of the PMQX scores as being:

Scores between	10-19	=	significantly untherapeutic attitude
Scores between	20-29	=	noticeably untherapeutic attitude
	30	=	minimally therapeutic attitude
Scores between	31-40	=	noticeably therapeutic attitude
Scores between	41-50	=	significantly therapeutic attitude

None of the sample scores in this study fall within the significantly untherapeutic attitude range, only three scores fall in the noticeably untherapeutic attitude range, and three scores in the minimally therapeutic range. The majority of responses thus fall within the noticeably or significantly therapeutic attitude range (96.87%). It may therefore be concluded that a large majority of the sample for this study display highly patient-centred attitudes.

Analysis of the PMQX data

This section of the study focuses on statistical analysis of the PMQX data with regard to a number of independent variables. The null hypothesis being tested is:

There are no significant differences in the PMQX scores in relation to the independent variables of sex, age, year of training, academic level of the course, branch studies being undertaken or educational institution.

Table 6.53 gives the Mann-Whitney test results regarding sex. There is a significant difference, in that the females in the sample are shown to have significantly higher patient-centred scores. There are no significant differences with regard to the academic level of the courses the sample are undertaking.

Table 6.53
Mann-Whitney scores by sex and academic level

	U Score	2-tailed probability
Gender	2102.5	0.0140*
Academic level	4384.0	0.0794

Table 6.54 shows no significant differences with regard to ages of the sample, the branch studies the sample are undertaking or the institution where the sample are taking their course. There is, however, a significant result in that students in their third year of training are shown to have significantly higher patient-centred scores.

Table 6.54
Chi-Square scores by age, year of training, branch studies and institution

	Chi-Square	Significance
Age	2.4018	0.4894
Year of training	7.1277	0.0275*
Branch studies	3.4896	0.3181
Institution	12.8832	0.2936

Comparisons of PMQX and SAQ scores

The final part of analysis of the results of this study relates to comparisons between the institutions' mean SAQ scores and student groups' mean PMQX scores. The null hypothesis to be tested is:

There are no significant differences between institutions' SAQ scores and student groups' PMQX scores.

Table 6.55 gives the Spearman Correlation Coefficients of the PMQX and SAQ scores, and there is no significant correlation between the two sets of scores. Therefore no statistical relationship can be demonstrated between institutions which are defined as being highly student-centred as and student groups from the same institutions who are defined as being highly patient-centred.

Table 6.55
Spearman correlation coefficient of PMQX and SAQ scores

Correlation coefficient	Significance
0.1965	0.540

The absence of any statistical relationship between the two sets of scores is also demonstrated in the scatter diagram given in figure 6.2.

Summary of the analysis of the PMQX

It has been shown in this section that the student nurses surveyed generally had high PMQX scores, which indicates markedly therapeutic attitudes. This is a reassuring result in terms of the implication this has for their behaviour in actual patient care situations.

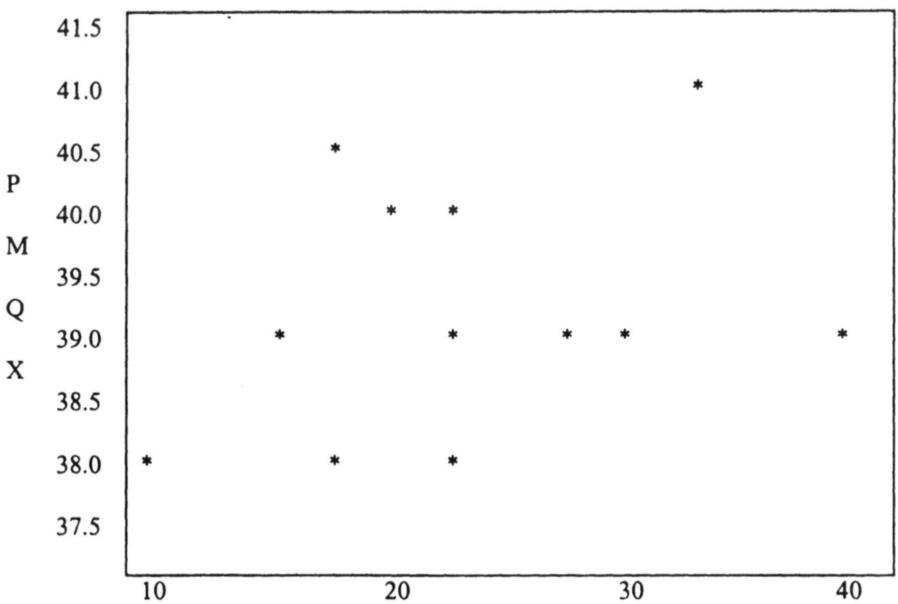

Figure 6.2 **Scatter diagram of correlations of PMQX and SAQ scores**

Statistical analysis shows that females in the sample and those in their third year of training had significantly higher PMQX scores. Whilst the results will be discussed further in the following chapter, possible explanations could be that females have greater tendencies to care which may be related to their biological child-bearing function and their customary social roles of child-rearing. That students in their third year of training have significantly higher scores, however, could be interpreted as meaning that appropriate patient-centred attitudes are learnt in pre-registration nurse education. This explanation therefore contradicts the interpretation that females are more caring due to inborn female abilities. The evidence in this study would seem to indicate that patient-centredness is an attitude that is learnt.

The final part of the data analysis fails to give any validity to one of the central focuses of this study in that no relationship can be demonstrated between measures of patient-centredness and student-centredness. However, whilst there is no statistical evidence of such a relationship, a number of important issues and relationships have been identified in previous sections of the data analysis. These will be key areas in the following chapter of this book, which is devoted to discussion of the findings of this study.

7 Discussion of the findings of the study

The aim of this chapter is to out–line the major findings of this study and to compare the results with relevant published literature. As related previously it should be noted that the literature review given in chapters two and three is given as the basis for subsequent development of the SAQ instrument and as such has not been amended or updated. A further aim of this chapter is therefore to examine recent and current published literature in regard of the research findings.

An intention of this study has been to explore relationships between how pre–registration student nurses are taught with attitudes to nursing care delivery. An emphasis, therefore, has been to demonstrate relationships between application of student–centred approaches to learning and teaching and patient–centred approaches to nursing care. Utilising role modelling theory as a theoretical framework, roles of nurse teachers are seen as being of pivotal importance. However, through use of methodological triangulation creation of a three dimensional picture has also been an aim. For example, there has been an intention to focus upon comparisons between nurse education institutionals' 'official' attitudes to student–centredness, to values and attitudes of nurse teachers, and student nurses to both student–centredness and patient–centredness.

The results of the study pertaining to the first research question

The first research question relates to attitudes of senior educational managers in educational institutions where pre–registration nurse training occurs regarding beliefs and concepts pertaining to student–centred learning and teaching and andragogy.

Student–centred learning and teaching as a dominant nursing educational philosophy

The high agreement responses to the majority of the SAQ statements gives verification to student–centred learning and teaching as an overtly dominant 'official' educational philosophy in pre–registration nurse education in England. These results give vindication to the basic framework of the SAQ as developed out of an initial review of the published literature. For example, self–directed, experiential, problem–solving learning and teaching are shown to be perceived as major dimensions of student–centredness.

That student–centred learning and teaching is exhorted as a 'correct' education philosophy in nurse education is shown in views expressed by a number of authors. For example, Beckett & Wall (1985), Burnard (1989a), Chally (1992), Goodall (1985), Jarvis (1992a), Jasper (1994), Richardson (1988), Rideout (1994) and Taylor (1993), all advocate student–centredness in nurse education programmes. However, whilst student–centred learning and teaching is thought by the majority to an inimitable approach to nurse education there are doubts expressed if this approach is an actuality. For example, Woodrow (1993) and Diekelmann (1993) relate that behaviourist practises are dominant in nurse education. Findings of this study give verification of high attitude agreement scores to the majority of dimensions of student–centred learning and teaching. However, there is no evidence of how these espoused beliefs are translated into actual learning and teaching interactions.

Andragogical tenets

The SAQ also gives evidence of positive attitudes regarding andragogical tenets. A number of authors advocate incorporating andragogical principles in nurse education (Neilsen 1992, Myles 1991 and Orr 1990). However, in recent literature there is some doubt expressed regarding the appropriateness of andragogical philosophy. For example, Darbyshire (1994), Platt (1988) and Woodrow (1993) question that andragogy is the same as student–centred learning and teaching. In a similar critique by Mezirow (1981) given in chapter 2, all argue that the basis tenets of andragogy are flawed because it differentiates between the learning processes of children and adults. Platt and Woodrow also relate that andragogy is directed towards 'labelling' adult learners as a homogeneous group and so ignores individuality in the teaching and learning process. For example, Platt states that it is wrong to assume all adults are capable of self–directiveness in the learning process.

Barriers to adopting referred teaching and learning philosophies

Significant results were obtained in the SAQ survey regarding independent context variables of class and cohort size. These results gives limited evidence that adopting student–centred learning and teaching in nurse education may be being adversely affected by large class and cohort sizes. There is a substantial body of literature emerging with regard to evaluation of Project 2000 style pre–registration nurse education (Elkan and Robinson 1995, Hallett et al 1995, Hamill 1995, Jasper 1994, Jones et al 1994, Perry 1990, Phillips 1994, Smith 1994 and Wilson–Barnett et al 1995). There is little reference to large cohort and class as apparent in some institutions surveyed and their impact on learning and teaching processes. However, Jones et al (1994) does relate that the size of Project 2000 cohorts makes the successful management of small tutorial groups 'extremely challenging'. Studdy et al

(1994) likewise relates organising small group teaching for skills training to be a difficult endeavour.

Key concepts of student–centred learning and teaching and andragogy

Identification of key concepts of student–centreness was an intention of the factor analysis of the SAQ data. Comparisons between the descriptive statistical analysis section of the SAQ data and the factor analysis gives interesting findings. For example, individuality in learning and teaching processes, through taking account of learning styles and learning preferences, and nurse teachers negotiating regarding the teaching and learning methods used, are unified together as a major factor. However, in the descriptive statistical section it is demonstrated that there are not strong agreement responses to any of these statements, nor to that of individualising learning through the use of contract learning. Therefore it may be concluded that there is evidence in this study of the centrality of meeting individual needs in student–centred learning and teaching. However, there is little evidence from the SAQ survey that educational practises designed to individualise the educational process are adhered to.

The results of the study pertaining to the second research question

The second research question pertains to what are values and perceptions of nurse teachers with regard to the concepts of student–centred learning and teaching and patient–centred care.

Consistencies between the SAQ data and the nurse teacher data were found in regards in beliefs regarding the three main dimensions of student–centredness, namely the importance self–directed, active, problem–solving teaching and learning.

Individual learning needs

Similarly to the SAQ data addressing individual learning needs were identified as a focal issue of student–centredness by the interviewees. However it can be seen as debatable if compliance to individual learning needs is being achieved. For example, in the data category pertaining to teaching and learning preferences whilst individuality was identified as being important it appear to be subsumed under student group learning and teaching preferences. Also there was very little evidence in the nurse teacher data of deployment of learning style inventories as a way of adapting teaching methods as appropriate for the learning styles of individual students.

Addressing individual needs of students through use of contract learning is also shown in all the data obtained not to be in widespread use. A number of authors give the value of contract learning as a method of identifying and meeting individual student needs (Carlisle 1991, Rideout 1994, Sutcliffe 1993). However, whilst some of the nurse teachers interviewed saw contract learning to be of use in specific situations most identified resourcing issues as precluding extensive use.

As with the SAQ data barriers to use of preferred teaching methods given by the interviewees gives explanation to why it is sometimes seen as difficult to address individual learning needs in nurse education programmes. For example, the lack of physical and human resources and large class sizes were identified as being problematical areas by the interviewees. Elkan and Robinson (1995) describe how the speed of implementation of Project 2000 courses resulted in initial problems. Jones et al (1995) and Studdy et al (1994) also relates difficulties regarding large cohort and class sizes. However the majority of the literature in respect of both diploma and degree level pre–registration courses does not address resourcing issues in a covert way.

It can therefore be shown in the first theme of the nurse teacher interviews as with the SAQ data, that there is general agreement with regard to some of the principles of student–centred learning and teaching. Individuality of learning needs and self–directed, active, problem–solving learning and teaching are seen as key concepts.

Teacher/student nurse power relationships

Analysis of data categories concerning andagogy and power relationships, however, calls into question how deeply embedded student–centred, andragogical philosophy is in nurse education in England. For example, number of interviewees thought pre–registration nurse education has a teacher–centred orientation with the power–base resting with teachers and institutions. Current practises of monitoring student attendance was also seen by some as contradictory to andragogical principles.

These findings are in accord with Brown's (1993) findings of how nurse teachers and students perceive power to operate in their relationships. For example, Brown found curriculum content as being totally controlled by teachers although students did have slightly more say over their learning methods.

Behaviourist learning theories

In other data categories of the nurse teacher interviews it was shown that behavioural learning theories and teaching methods were seen as appropriate in certain situations. A balanced approach regarding application of learning and teaching theories was preferred by a number of interviewees.

Generally it can be concluded there is no evidence of the primacy of any one learning theory and its applicability to pre–registration nurse education. For example, whilst there is no evidence that vindicates the beliefs of Diekelmann (1993), Farmer (1992) and Woodrow (1993) that nurse education has a predominantly behaviourist focus. Equally there is no evidence that student–centred, adult learning and teaching principles are a dominant educational philosophy in pre–registration nurse education in England. However, as with the SAQ data, how the espoused beliefs and attitudes of the interviewees are translated into educational encounters is beyond the scope of this study.

The role of the nurse teacher – desirable teacher qualities

The second major theme of the nurse teacher interviews was the role of the nurse teacher. Desirable teacher qualities were seen as being a facilitator of learning, a resource person and an up–to–date expert. All of these qualities are identified by Crotty (1993) in a study of the current role of nurse teachers in respect of Project 2000 diploma courses as being of importance.

The role of the nurse teacher – personal tutor systems

A major dimension of the role of nurse teachers can be identified in that of as being a 'support person'. Conversely to findings discussed previously, personal tutor systems were identified by a number of interviewees as an institutional mechanism designed to address individual student needs. A number of studies demonstrate that support of students is an important facet of the role of nurse teachers (Cohen 1993, Komorita et al 1991, Nelms et al 1993, Paterson and Crawford 1994 and Wiseman 1994). Whilst, for example, Paterson and Crawford identify that 'knowing the student' is of vital importance few studies identify how support and individualisation of learning needs can be articulated in a formal systematic way.

Phillips (1994) does, however, describe the personal tutor dimension of the nurse teachers' role. Phillips relates how concepts of 'personal tutors' has evolved with little apparent active planning. Advantages of personal tutor systems are seen as providing individual support especially with regard to academic guidance. This guidance is seen as being needed following large impersonal lectures as sometimes deployed in Project 2000 diploma courses. However, Phillips also identifies problems of achieving the right balance between a professional–friendship type personal tutor model and over–involved, over–dependent type model.

The description of personal tutor systems given by Phillips (1994) can be shown to correspond to the data obtained from the nurse teacher interviews conducted. For example, the majority of those interviewed thought their institution has an effective personal tutor system which supported and provided for the individual student learning needs. Academic and pastoral support were identified as key features of the role. However, if the pastoral support given to students complies to an over–involved, over–dependent type model described by Phillips (1994) cannot be demonstrated.

The role of the nurse teacher – clinical dimensions

Crotty (1993) identifies a major preoccupation of nurse teachers in her study was that of their clinical role. Similarly in this study a significant number of data categories emerged appertaining to the clinical role of the nurse teacher especially with regard to nurse teachers acting as role models for students when learning about nursing.

There is an abundance of published literature regarding clinical roles of nurse teachers (Acton et al 1992, Baillie 1994, Clifford 1993, Charlesworth et al 1992, Crotty 1993, Fawcett and McQueen 1994, and Jinks 1991). Many of the findings of this study are congruent with the published literature. For example, Clifford and

Charlesworth et al relate how following the demise of the clinical teacher the role has been not been replaced. Clifford and Crotty describe how nurse teachers do not see their role as teaching 'hands on nursing' but acting as a liaison person between education and practice. Jinks also describes how an important function of nurse teachers in clinical areas is to enable student relate theory to practice. Whilst Crotty and Baillie identify a strong commitment by the nurse teachers in their studies to clinical liaison roles or clinical link systems, Acton et al relates there is insufficient motivation from nurse education hierarchies for nurse teachers clinical proficiency to be maintained. Clifford and Fawcett and McQueen also state that the major barrier to maintaining effective clinical link systems are constraints of time, with classroom activities being seen as a priority.

Nurse teachers as role models for student nurses learning about clinical practice

In the nurse teacher data of this study it was found whilst maintaining clinical link and clinical teaching commitments was difficult the majority felt they were able to maintain their clinical skills on a personal basis. However, they did not see themselves as acting as credible role models for student nurses learning about clinical practice. Hence it may be concluded that maintaining clinical proficiently is viewed as a personal endeavour and divorced form the pragmatic issues surrounding clinical teaching and formalised clinical link systems. Also there is little evidence that nurse teachers in this study see themselves as acting as role models for student learning about nursing. 'Nursing' was interpreted by all the interviewees in a practical context. It was said by a number of interviewees that because students do not see them as practising nurses they are not role models. Clinical staff, students' own peers and patients were seen as being the most important role models for students learning about nursing.

There is only a limited amount of literature in respect of role imitation by student nurses of nurse teacher behaviour. However, Davies (1993) found similarly to the nurse teacher data, that important role models for students were students' own peers, and supervisory nurses in the clinical areas. Nelms et al (1993) in a North American context, however, found that patient care given by teachers and observed by students, was an important influence on student attitudes to care delivery. The validity of comparisons to an American study is, however, dubious because of the very different approaches taken to practical nurse training.

Patient–centred care

The final data theme of the nurse teacher interviews relates to patient–centred care. In accord with the literature given in chapter 3 the nursing process was identified by the interviewees as the most desirable way of delivering nursing care. Negative features of the nursing process were also identified. Not least of these features is that it is poorly used by clinical practitioners. The nursing process was, however, identified as an appropriate framework for articulating often personal values about how nursing care should be approached. These values correspond to humanistic philosophy as also discussed in chapter 3. Recognition of the individual and their humaness were cardinal features of these personal values systems. A data category also emerged that patients should be involved in decision making concerning their care.

Patient–empowerment

The concept of patient–empowerment is the subject of many current social policy initiatives. For example, Cohen (1994) examines patient–empowerment through introduction of the Patients' Charter. In a similar context Wilson (1992) also examines the role of self–help groups. Jewell (1994) in an empirical study, however, explores patient participation and what it means for nurses. Using primary nurses as a sample Jewell found patient–centredness was of central importance and patients were viewed as potential collaborators in care decisions. However, similarly to the data in this study, it was shown that it was seen as appropriate if patients wished 'to opt out'. Also some patients' poor mental health made their participation difficult. Thus individual assessment regarding patient participation is of central importance. Similarly Hogston (1995) found addressing patients individual needs of key issue and that nurses in the study defined quality patient care in terms of patient satisfaction.

Care and care–giving

Patient satisfaction or how patients define important caring behaviours of nurses has been the subject of a number of studies. For example, Price (1993) found in a study of parents perceptions of quality nursing care that competent technical function was a basic expectation. This finding is similar to the studies of Larson (1984, 1986, and 1987). However, Price found that elements of 'quality care' was the interest, concern and affection nurses demonstrated.

Caring for patients was seen by the interviewees in this study as an important nursing value. Care as a central feature of nursing was explored in chapter 3. The emotional, loving dimension of care giving was compared to a wider moral dimension of recognition as patients as persons. However, more recent literature has questioned the nature of care in a nursing context. For example, Champion (1991) relates that care may mean 'concern for' but also 'acting for'. Thus as a concept care can enhances patient dependency. Champion states that nursing care should be about patient self–determination and helping a person onwards. 'Being with' but not necessarily 'doing for'.

Caffery (1994) and Colman (1993) also identify problems with care as a key concept in nursing. For example, it is stated by Colman that some enter a career in nursing to achieve personal goals of love and respect of others and therefore are over–carers in a nursing role. A co–dependent caring model between nurses and patients is hypothesised. Similarly Caffrey sees dependent caring as feeding nurses' self–esteem. Altruistic self–sacrifice models of care have the potential to undermine patient autonomy. Colman also sees the public as over–dependent and have an unconscious wish to remain so. Therefore it is seen there is an inherent tension in nursing between those who are over–carers and those who strive for patient autonomy and independence. There is also a potential tension between a public wish to be dependent in nursing care situations and a nursing aim to promote independence.

Caring for patients and caring for students

This analysis of care may be compared to the data of the final category of the nurse teachers interviews where paradigms of caring for students and caring for patients are given. The majority saw care for patients as a being different to care for students. For example, both the quantity and quality was seen to differ. However, based on a number of examples of 'caring for students' given by the intervewees it can be hypothesised that some may perceive themselves as over–carers in both patient care and student care situations. As with other findings it is not possible to demonstrate how these beliefs are translated in actual 'student care' situations.

It may be concluded from the nurse teacher interviews that concepts of individualism, humanism, empowerment and care are key factors in both patient–centred and student–centred learning. These findings correspond with the trend in the current literature to discuss student–centred learning and teaching within a individualistic, humanistic, caring and empowering framework (Bevis and Murray 1990, Chally 1992, Cohen 1993, Dawson 1994, Diekelmann 1990, Paterson and Crawford 1994, Schmieding 1993, Tanner 1990).

The results of the study pertaining to the third research question

The third research question relates to pre–registration student nurses' perceptions of student–centred learning and teaching.

Student nurse perceptions of student–centred learning and teaching

How the student nurses surveyed perceived student–centred learning and teaching is shown broadly to compare with both the SAQ and interviewee data. Being treated as an individual and as an adult is identified as being of major importance. However, a key feature of the student nurse data is also being in receipt of effective and appropriate teaching.

Effective teaching

Eason and Corbett (1991), Fong and McCauley (1993), MacLeod (1995) and Schumann (1990) refer to good quality teaching as an important issue for student nurses. For example, MacLeod distinguishes being learning and being well taught. Learning is seen as a deeper understanding through student involvement, whereas being well taught is experiencing a structure for learning. A primary goal of successfully completing the course through acquiring appropriate knowledge was central for the students in MacLeod's study. The outcome or product of teaching and learning is shown in data analysis pertaining to a number of questions in the student nurse survey to be an important factor also for respondents in the present study. However, the nurse teacher data demonstrates an emphasis on the process of teaching and learning rather than the outcome.

Self–directed learning

Positive attitudes to self–directed learning can be shown in all sets of data in this study. However, the nurse teachers see some basic knowledge of topic areas as a prerequisite for self–directed learning by students. Also they appeared to under–estimate students' self–directed learning abilities, whilst students were shown to feel that support, guidance and feedback from teachers is not always adequate. Findings of the SAQ survey and the nurse teacher interviews are in accord with a general recommendation in the literature of this approach. Prociuk (1990) and St Claire and Brillhart (1990) state a need for nurses to be self–directed learners. However, the student nurse data in this study reveals some potential disparity with certain findings reported in the literature.

Burnard and Morrison (1992), Demirbag and Ridenour (1995), Hamill (1995) and MacLeod (1995) identify that self–directed learning is not a highly preferred learning method of student nurses. Burnard and Morrison found that, whilst 75% of the student nurses in their survey saw self–directed learning as a preferred learning method, this could be compared with over 93% of nurse teachers surveyed. Demirbag and Ridenour similarly found that self–pacing was the least preferred learning method identified by nurses in their study. Hamill also reports that student stress was exacerbated by too much self–directed learning and confusion regarding assignment guidelines. Finally, MacLeod found that students were dismayed at the need for self–direction and wanted teachers to give explicit, concrete expectations of learning outcomes.

Findings of the present study in replies to questions directly relating to self–directed learning and also in replies to other questions does give evidence that self–directed learning is a learning and teaching method commonly used in the students' course. Also there is evidence that students can identify positive learning benefits from self–directed learning and it is a preferred method of learning for some students. However, there is no evidence that self–directed learning is highly ranked amongst preferred learning methods for the student sample in its entirety. Indeed at a later point in this chapter it will be shown that more formal didactic learning methods are preferred. In addition it was reported in the data that stress can be caused through students not having enough support, guidance and feedback regarding self–directed study.

Development of self–directed learning skills

The responses to the question posed to the student nurses regarding development of self–directed learning skills demonstrate a significant difference from both the SAQ and interview data. The students are shown to feel that such skills are not taught on their courses. Those who felt that such skills had been addressed referred to development of study skills. Comparison of these findings to other research findings shows a number of authors advocating 'learning to learn' type programmes as a part of developing self–directed learning skills (Jarvis 1992b, Jones et al 1994, Schmidt and Fisher 1993). However, an empirical study by Wiley (1983) establishes little difference in the students' ability to direct their own learning in samples who had undertaken such a programmes and those who had not. As shown in the student data in the present study, it could therefore be concluded that individual motivation to learn and self–teaching of these skills are perhaps equally important issues.

Experiential learning

Experiential and active learning are shown in all the data sets to be important features of student–centred learning and also of the courses the student sample are undertaking. However, whilst the nurse teachers interpreted experiential learning as occurring mainly in the classroom, a large majority of students related it to learning in clinical settings. These findings are in accord to the findings of Burnard (1992a), where it was found students felt they learned most about nursing from working in clinical settings. It was also reported by the students in the present study that more clinical practice was needed on their courses. Again Elkan and Robinson (1995) and Jones et al (1994) reported similar concerns expressed by students in their studies.

A area of experiential learning identified in the chapter 2 was reflection on nursing practice. Reflective practice was shown in the SAQ survey and nurse teacher interviews to accrue strong values. This is congruent with current interest nurse educationalists have in the subject. For example, Darbyshire (1993), James and Clarke (1994), Lauder (1994), Newell (1994) and Reid (1993) advocate reflective nursing practice. Darbyshire also sees reflection on practice as giving both 'freedom to think' and 'empowerment to think'. It is through 'empowerment to think' that Darbyshire identifies that changes to ritualised, non–individualised and impersonal nursing practice will occur.

There is, therefore, some discord between the sets of data in that reflective practice is not mentioned by any of the students in response to the question regarding active learning and infrequently in responses to other questions. It will be shown at a later point in this discussion that informal group discussions are a preferred learning method. It may be that reflection on practice is incorporated into these sessions. However, it cannot be shown that the current interest and importance invested by nurse educationalists in reflection on practice is replicated by the values of the student nurses surveyed.

Problem–solving learning

Comparisons of findings of the data sets pertaining to problem–solving learning again demonstrate diverse responses. All the data sets demonstrate general positive attitudes to these skills as part of student–centred learning and teaching. Frequently it can be demonstrated that these skills are related to use of the nursing process. However, the student nurses are shown to generally feel that there is not enough teaching regarding problem–solving. Comparisons with students' feelings that there is not enough clinical practice in their courses may be made. So, for example, not only do the students feel that there is not enough clinical practice in their courses but also that there is not enough teaching in their institutions regarding the skills needed for clinical practice.

Creedy and Hand (1994) identify that problem–based learning employs approaches to teaching and learning that develop meaningful links between theory and practice. A problem–solving approach is defined as management of real–life difficulties through application of appropriate knowledge. A small number of students in the present sample do mention problem–solving in nursing studies context and the use of case study material as a basis for developing problem–solving skills. However, generally the data would seem to indicate that students surveyed perceive this to be an under–addressed area.

Learning preferences expressed by the student nurses

It was shown earlier that taking account of individual learning needs and preferences is of key importance in how student–centred learning and teaching is defined. However, both the SAQ and interviewee data give evidence of difficulties in achieving individuality in the learning and teaching process. It is shown in this study that the learning method most frequently mentioned by the students is that of lectures. However, generally a large number of teaching methods were mentioned, with individual respondents identifying an inter–mix of methods.

A number of studies show students nurses to prefer didactic teaching methods. Burnard and Morrison (1992), demonstrate that students in their sample preferred teacher–centred approaches, whereas the nurse teachers studied preferred student–centred approaches. Similarly Demirbag and Ridenour (1995) show a preference for didactic teaching methods by nurses in their study. However Vaughan's (1990) study gives contrary findings to those of Burnard and Morrison. Jones et al (1994) also identify that the students in their study demonstrate a preference for working in small groups, with one–to–one tutorials being highly valued.

It may be concluded from the results of the present study and also from the findings of other studies that student nurses cannot be considered to be a homogeneous group in terms of their learning preferences. An inter–mix of methods and interesting, relevant and stimulating teaching is important. Therefore application of a learning theory which implies one method or a group of similar methods is inappropriate.

Nursing skills training

A teaching method that is identified in responses to the question regarding preferred teaching methods, and also in responses to other questions, is nursing skills training. It was shown in the nurse teacher interviews that skills training emerged as a discrete data category. Whilst it was shown that certain skills are being taught in the classroom in some institutions, generally it was thought that this is currently an under–addressed area. Similarly a small proportion of responses in the student nurse data identify a preference for skills training and the need for more skills training.

Elkan and Robinson (1995) and Hamill (1995) identify the students in their studies as feeling unconfident and incompetent regarding practical skills. Bjork (1995) in a Scandinavian context relates that internationally there appears to be a lack of interest in how and if students acquire the necessary practical skills central to therapeutic care. It is said by Bjork that the practical aspects of nursing actions have been 'isolated' and defined as psychomotor skills. Bjork states that discourse on the elements of nursing care needs to take heed of patients' perceptions of good nursing care and attention needs to be given to the physical and practical aspects of care delivery. These are similar to conclusions drawn earlier in this chapter which identified areas of discord between nurses' and patients' perceptions of what constitutes effective nursing care.

The work of Studdy et al (1994) reflects the concern of nurse educationalists with clinical skills development and proposes a teaching model and schedule for skills development. Difficulties of students observing, acquiring and practising clinical skills are identified. Changes in practice are seen by Studdy et al as reasons for these difficulties. An increased emphasis on community care, day care and outpatient teaching, with the concomitant increase in dependency and throughput of in–patients, makes it increasingly difficult for students to be taught the appropriate skills needed for practice.

Student nurse self–esteem

The findings of this study in respect to whether students in the sample are treated as adults and as individuals are generally of a positive nature. Just under three quarters of the sample felt they had been treated as an adult by the majority of people they had come into contact with whilst on their course. Similarly over half the sample felt they were treated as an individual. However, 'knowing' students through use of individuals' names is identified as a problem for some teachers and students. Failure to know students has been shown to be a possible consequence of large group sizes in nurse education programmes.

Negative responses of the students in this study may be compared to the research of Theis (1988). Theis states that unethical teaching behaviour relates to lack of respect for students through insensitivity toward learners, and ridiculing and belittling teaching behaviour. Some teacher and clinical staff behaviours can be inferred from the data to conform to Theis's unethical teaching model. However, there is no evidence regarding other dimensions identified by Theis concerning lack of respect for patients and violation of justice, such as, for example, showing favouritism, prejudice or unfair testing and grading practices.

Generally it can be concluded that addressing student individuality and self–esteem is felt by the students in the sample to be reasonably satisfactory. This may be compared with the SAQ and nurse teacher data where, although valuing these concepts, doubts were expressed if they were conformed to in educational practices. However, findings of other studies are shown to be contrary to findings of the present study. For example, Hamill (1995) reports that the students studied did not feel they were treated as adults. Similarly McFall (1995), from a student nurse perspective, states that students are expected to behave in a child–like role.

The importance of teaching behaviour for student nurses' self–esteem was discussed in the initial review of the literature. It was hypothesized that self–concept and confidence in clinical abilities were integrally linked. However, the results of the study demonstrate that clinical practice and clinical skills are areas of concern for both students and teachers in the study. Indications are that the majority of students surveyed feel they are treated in ways that are likely to develop their self–esteem.

Influential people in the student nurses' learning about nursing

One of the final questions in the student nurse survey relates to influential people in how students learn about nursing. Whilst a substantial number of student responses concern the influence of clinical staff and clinical experiences, the most frequently mentioned group of people were nurse teachers. These findings are in direct contrast to the nurse teacher interview data, where nurse teachers' influence appeared to be under–estimated.

These findings are contrary to the findings of studies of the socialisation of nursing students. Whilst a number of studies report that ward learning environments are at times unsatisfactory (Greenwood 1993, Hamill 1995, Orr 1990), others give the most important socialising influence as clinical staff and clinical experiences (Baillie 1994, Hallett et al 1995, Melia 1984). Melia, for example, in a classic study of the socialisation of student nurses' reports that permanent ward staff and other student nurses appeared to be the most significant people in the students studied perceptions. Melia's study was, however, conducted prior to the implementation of Project 2000 courses. It is hypothesed by Chandler (1991) that Project 2000 courses' emphasis on the theoretical base of nursing, the move into higher education establishments, and the supernumerary status of students in clinical areas would change how, and from whom, nursing is learnt. It would seem that the evidence in the present study would give credence to the beliefs of Chandler, in that, whilst clinical staff and students own peers are still important influences, nurse teachers are seen as the most significant people to the students surveyed.

The results of the study pertaining to the fourth research question

The final research question concerns how student nurse PMQX scores compare to their institutions' SAQ scores. It was shown in the previous chapter that there are no significant relationships between the two scores. Therefore one of the central premises of this study cannot overtly be demonstrated. It cannot be shown that, if students are taught in a student–centred fashion by nurse teachers, these concepts will be translated into care delivery through the adoption of patient–centred attitudes.

The findings of the PMQX survey does, however, give some reassuring results. Only 3 students in the sample are shown to have untherapeutic attitudes, also third year students in the sample are shown to have significantly higher scores. It is concluded, therefore, that patient–centredness is an attitude that can be developed during nurse training programmes.

These results are similar to those of the author of the PMQX who found that a very small proportion of student nurses studied had untherapeutic attitudes (Rolfe 1993b). Sheahan (1991) also found the students in his study to enter nursing with a person–centred attitude. However, similarly to Sheahan's study, Rolfe's sample only comprised of students who were at an early stage in their training, therefore comparisons between measurements of attitudes of students at different points of training are not possible. Seed (1994) does, however, state that findings of her study indicate that student nurses' perceptions follow along a continuum. During occupational socialisation, the students Seed studied, moved from 'seeing patients' to 'seeing people'. Implicit in Seed's findings is that student adopt a more individualistic attitude to patient care as they progress through their course.

The findings of the present study and similar studies may, however, be compared to those of Burnard and Morrison (1991). It was found that students in their study were more client–centred than were trained nurses. This illustrates similar points made in this chapter that attitude analysis is only valid at a given point in time. Therefore no verification can be given that attitudes of patient–centredness in the students studied will be displayed in their current or future nursing practice.

It was found that females in the student nurse sample had significantly higher PMQX scores. It could therefore be inferred that females have greater tendencies to care, which may be related to child–bearing and their customary social role of child–rearing. As a consequence of these roles, nurturing and caring are identified as common expectations of female stereotypical behaviour. A number of authors identify relationships between nurturing and care–giving in a nursing context (Dingwall et al 1988, Jinks 1993, Morrison 1992, Savage 1987, Webb 1986). Of central concern, however, is how care in a nursing context is defined.

Individualism, humanism, care and empowerment

The idea of treating people as people, which also incorporates humanistic values, has been a recurrent issue in this study. Earlier discussion of care as a nursing concept has shown that empathetic 'being with' patients is a cardinal feature of good nursing care. However, an altruistic self–sacrifice model has been shown as being inappropriate for professional nursing caring behaviour. Therefore whilst nurses may care for patients as people, this does not necessarily imply that they help or 'do for people'. A crucial distinction between a nurturing caring model and a nursing caring model is helping or 'doing for' as compared to promoting mastery over one's own life.

Patient empowerment gives freedom to participate in self–caring on a continuum. The continuum can range from self–care and independence to a nurse–care dependent model. As described by Orem (1980), a primary nursing goal is to move patients, whenever possible, from dependence to maximum independence. It has, however, been shown earlier that patient empowerment may be at odds with the desires and wishes of individual patients and indeed the population as a whole.

Patient empowerment is, however, difficult not merely because of possible conflict between patient– and nurse–desired outcomes of care delivery. Gibson (1991) and Skelton (1994) report that self–care is a currently favoured political ideology in the United Kingdom. Thus moral and social obligations are dimensions of the sick–role on a micro level. True empowerment is not, however, just about self–care. In its wider dimensions it is a genuine hand–over of power through providing access to information, participation in resource allocation and health care decision–making at a macro level.

Structural elements in society, such as existing professional and governmental power groups, are therefore potential barriers to true patient–empowerment. Nursing is not an autonomous professional group, for example, it has constraints on action placed upon it by more powerful professional groups such as medicine and management. Nevertheless it is thought that nursing needs to take a revolutionary rather than reformist approach to care delivery. Thus empowerment through nursing actions entails a process of helping individuals, groups and communities to develop a critical awareness of the root causes of their problems and a readiness to act on this information. Patient advocacy may therefore on occasions be a central feature of nursing intervention.

Notions of caring for patients and caring for students has been a central theme of this study. Caring for students has been articulated through examination of the currently favoured student–centred teaching and learning philosophy and andragogical ideology and a research hypothesis which has role model imitation as a focal feature. Individualist and humanistic underpinning of these approaches to learning and teaching have been identified as of key importance both in the findings of this study and of similar studies.

Paterson and Crawford (1994) give an analysis of caring in nurse education. They identify that definitions of care in an educational context are rarely given in the literature and it is assumed that caring skills of nursing practice are simply transferred to the arena of nurse education. Paterson and Crawford conjecture that if one can care as a nurse, one can care for students as an educator. Generally therefore they suggest that caring for students is a moral imperative of nurse educators. Paterson and Crawford, however, relate that caring for students is not something that is 'done for students' but is part of the context in which students are taught.

The context in which student nurses are taught must obviously include observing and experiencing caring behaviours. In the present study, clinical roles of nurse teachers and how students learn about clinical practice are shown to be important caring experiences for students. However, as described previously in terms of care for patients, care for students is not defined as compliance to an ethic of selfless giving. It is defined as satisfactory provision of professional nursing caring experiences, transmission of appropriate knowledge for nursing practice, and finally, through effective educational practises, equipping student nurses with the skills to be autonomous in identifying and fulfilling their future learning needs.

A further dimension of caring for students can be shown in another key finding of the present study, which is that teachers recognise students as worthwhile and unique, with individual needs and attributes. It is acknowledged that 'knowing' students in a meaningful way has been shown in this study to be a problematic area for students and teachers. However, a key feature of caring for students is thought to be 'knowing individual learning needs' and provision of appropriate teaching and learning activities to meet these needs.

These definitions of caring for students are similar to those given in literature pertaining to student empowerment. An important feature of student empowerment is described by Diekelmann (1990) as development and enablement to think critically through use of humanistic educational approaches. Through empowerment, students are able to critically analyse nursing practice and, where needed, instigate changes in care delivery. Similarly Cohen (1993) considers that an academic environment which promotes self–knowledge and self–esteem is an equally important dimension of student nurse empowerment.

The importance of nurse teachers to students' learning about nursing has been been demonstrated in this study. However, also identified is the fact that teacher interviewees generally feel unhappy regarding their clinical teaching role. A further question in this study is therefore whether nurse teachers can transmit care values effectively if they lack competence as a nurse. Is role modelling or effective teaching in an caring, humanistic, empowering framework the central issue in how student nurses learn about nursing practice?

Role imitation

Role imitation is described in chapter 3 as part of a social learning theory which may be defined as learning from other people through the mechanisms of reinforcement, observation and role modelling. Role imitation as part of this general theory is copying behaviours of significant others. Important role models for students learning about nursing were hypothesised at the beginning of this study to be nurse teachers. Whilst a number of significant others can be identified in the findings, the central importance of nurse teachers can be verified. However, the part that concepts of role imitation has in student nurses' learning about nursing is less clear.

It is evident that the majority of teachers studied do not see themselves as credible clinical role models. It is less clear, however, how the students view their teachers as clinical role models. Questions posed to the students were directed towards who were the most influential people for them in learning about nursing. Neither role models nor nursing practice were mentioned. It could be hypothesised that questions directly related to role models in clinical practice may have elicited more responses with regard to clinical staff. However, the results of this study would seem to indicate that role imitation of nurse teachers' clinical nursing behaviour is not an important variable in terms of how students learn about nursing. In view of the importance of the critical thinking abilities required for effective nurse practice the unquestioning mimicking of behaviour, appropriate or otherwise, in clinical setting is also probably an incongruous model for learning about nursing.

Evidence of caring and empowerment of the student nurses studied

Is there evidence to suggest that caring for students, and so empowering them, in an nurse education context, is of key importance? Generally the students surveyed demonstrated positive responses regarding learning and teaching practises. It would also appear that use of a single learning theory to structure learning experiences of student nurses is neither practised nor desirable from both teacher and student perspectives. Some of the students' negative responses and problems related to discrete areas of teaching and learning strategies indicate some improvements to the teaching and learning environments of the students studied are needed. However, positive indications of the self–esteem of students coupled with the generally high PMQX scores, implies that the students are reasonably satisfied with their learning environment and are developing appropriate attitudes to nursing care delivery. There is, therefore, a reasonable amount of evidence that the students studied are cared for by nurse teachers.

It may, therefore, finally be concluded that effective learning and teaching practises are more important issue in this study than role imitation

Limitations of the study

These general conclusions should, however, be tempered by the limitations of the study. Issues surrounding the reliability of the findings relate to the measurement instruments used. It has been demonstrated that the pilot study information regarding both the SAQ and PMQX instruments indicate reasonable evidence of the reliability of the measurement tools. However, further use of both scales would give greater reassurances regarding their reliability. Likewise greater evidence of the internal consistency of the SAQ and PMQX would be obtained through use in further studies.

Issues surrounding the validity of the results centre on measurement of attitudes. It has been stated at a number of points in the study that attitude measurement is only valid at a given point of time. Therefore measurement of attitudes cannot be used to predict future behaviour. Furthermore, because relatively small sample groups have been used for all sections of the research, justification for making generalisations from findings is questionable. Thus whilst inferences to other populations can be made, the findings of this study are only directly applicable to the sample groups used.

An issue in this study is the sampling procedures. For example, through use of mean institutional SAQ scores it is thought negative attitudes to the subject areas of the study were more likely to be identified. However, it is acknowledged that the high degree of compliance obtained from all the sample groups may have adversely affected this sampling objective. For instance, the nurse teacher interviewees were in effect volunteers. Therefore bias could be a feature of some of the data collected. For example, as 'volunteers' and through expressing a willingness to take part in the study, the nurse teachers interviewed may not represent the 'typical' views of nurse teachers. They may have been asked to 'volunteer' as they were perceived suitable persons to maintain the institution's public image. Similarly access to student groups was outside the control of the researcher. Therefore, as access was arranged by the individual institutions, it could be that the student samples are not representative of 'the average nursing student' either in the institution or nationally.

The research methodological framework may finally be seen to present potential problems. For example, Dootson (1995) and Dzurec and Abraham (1993) discuss the difficulties of linking quantitative and qualitative research in methodological triangulation. The strengths of this approach lie in giving a multi–faceted picture of research findings. Also the validity of findings is increased as one method's weaknesses are counter–balanced by the strengths of the other methods used. However it is recognised, as Dootson states, that there is a need to identify the dominant philosophical research paradigm which underpins a study. In this context the greater emphasis in the present study is the general survey approach taken.

Ethical considerations

Polit and Hungler (1991) state that the most fundamental ethical principle in research is the maxim of 'doing no harm'. Clearly, exposing research participants to experiences that could injury, disable, or cause death are not of relevance to this study. However, causing undue distress is a potential hazard of any research which involves researcher–participant interactions and clearly could be a feature of the study.

Exploitation of vulnerable groups, confidentiality and informed consent are other ethical principles which need to be examined with regard to this study. The student samples could be considered to be vulnerable groups. Participation in the study as part of the students' normal course timetable could make them vulnerable in a 'captive audience' sense. Confidentiality regarding some potentially sensitive issues discussed with the nurse teachers could also be identified as a further area where adhering to ethical principles is important. An example of issues surrounding informed consent is whether student and teacher participants should have been informed of the institutional selection procedure. A potential ethical dilemma was whether or not to reveal that institutions had a low or high SAQ scores.

It can be shown that all the relevant information regarding the study was given to all participants in advance letters and written information supplied on the data collection instruments. Additional reassurances were also given by the researcher at the point of data collection. The approach adopted was of honesty in responding to all questions asked. However, it was found that such questions were rarely asked either by the nurse teachers or student nurses.

Particular care was taken with regard to the student nurse samples. Although it was envisaged at the beginning of the research that permission would need to be sought from the individual institutions' ethics committees, surprisingly this was not necessary for any of the student groups. Careful explanation of the study and an emphasis on the voluntary nature of their participation was therefore a precursor of all the data collection sessions. However, apart from some members of one of the pilot group samples, no student refused to take part in the study. It can therefore be concluded that elements of either Milgram's (1974) 'compliance to a figure in authority' or the Hawthorne effect in which, 'compliance rates increase because of the interest the researcher is showing' (Roethlisberger and Dickson 1939) are features of the student nurse data collection sessions. Whilst it is impossible to be sure (and it is acknowledged that probably both elements are in part reasons for the high student compliance rate) researcher observations were that the students generally enjoyed completing the questionnaire. The first part seemed to give them opportunity to air their problems to a 'neutral' person. The PMQX section was seen as a test of their nursing ability and most appeared to want to achieve 'good marks'. Indeed a number of students asked if the researcher would forward their 'marks' to them.

A noticeable omission, however, from study in retrospect was the lack of use of consent forms. Whilst it can be stated that all moral and ethical principles have been adhered to, greater evidence could have been given by the inclusion of documentary evidence of consenting participation in the study. However, perhaps more importantly, the use of consent forms might have enforced particularly to the student groups that participation was entirely voluntary and that no sanctions would be taken against non–participants.

8 Conclusions and recommendations

Generally the study described in this book is seen as contributing to knowledge surrounding the theory:practice divide in nurse education. Effective integration of theory and practice is of obvious importance to nurse education programmes, however, it has been shown that the subject area is multi–faceted. This book has examined one dimension of this conundrum, namely use student–centred learning and teaching methods in nurse education and their interrelationships with patient–centred nursing care.

The findings of the study described would suggest that there are important interrelationships between caring for students and caring for patients. Whilst a direct relationship cannot be demonstrated through significant correlations between SAQ and PMQX scores a number of interesting findings have been given. A summary of the findings of the study and implications for future provision of pre–registration nurse education programmes is given in the following section.

Summary of the findings

There are a number of important findings given in this book which include conclusions drawn from the literature review, which indicate that teaching and learning methods used in nurse education is an under–researched area. The desirability of many of the philosophies and teaching and learning methods used cannot be verified through empirical research evidence. The need generally to conduct more research is clear if nurse education is to lay claims to having a research base to teaching and learning methods utilised in nurse education programmes.

The overall agreement scores in the SAQ survey suggests that student–centred learning and teaching and adherence to andragogical principles are dominant, overt values in pre–registration nurse education in England. Analysis of the nurse teacher and student nurse data, however, suggests that use of a variety of teaching methods which are stimulating and interesting, and which do not comply to use of a single learning theory is appropriate. Again further research is needed to give evidence to the validity of teaching and learning methods used by nurse teachers.

The SAQ data analysis gives a number of significant results. For example, the significant result regarding andragogical principles and those institutions conducting pre–Project 2000 courses is in accord with the published literature, which suggests that traditional nurse training programmes are teacher–centred. However, compliance to a progressive model of nurse education and by implication, incorporation student–centred learning methods, is called into question when other significant results of the SAQ data analysis are considered, namely those pertaining to class and cohort sizes. Large class and cohort sizes are identified as barriers to articulation of student–centred teaching and learning philosophies. These findings are of particular significance to the future resourcing of pre–registration nurse education. Smaller class sizes, adequate teaching accommodation and employment of more nurse teachers are areas which need to be addressed.

The factor analysis of the SAQ data demonstrates that individuality in meeting learning needs is a major underpinning concept of how student–centred learning is perceived by respondents in the study. Individuality was also found to be an important concept with regard to patient–centred nursing care in the views of the nurse teacher interviewees.

Whilst individuality in meeting the learning needs of students was identified as important by the nurse teachers interviewed, other findings of the data analysis show that tailoring teaching to take account of individual learning needs, is perceived as difficult, for similar reasons given in analysis of the SAQ data. Barriers to 'knowing' students in a meaningful way are again identified as being problematic against a back–drop of inadequate resources and large class sizes. Use of learning style inventories and contract learning in order to meet individual learning needs were identified as not in wide–spread use. However, personalising learning for students was seen as being facilitated through personal tutor systems. Given the apparent importance of personal tutor systems and the fact that it is an under–researched area, the need for more investigations into the subject area is evident.

A major concern of the teachers interviewed was that of their clinical role. Most of the interviewees thought maintaining their clinical competence as being addressed through personal endeavours, and largely divorced from the pragmatic issues surrounding clinical teaching and clinical link systems. Again the whole issue of nurse teachers' clinical roles warrants further investigation. There is also a need for nursings' professional bodies to consider policies which identify and prescribe what the clinical role of nurse teachers should be. This would give the lead for individual educational institutions to create an environment which values and facilitates nurse teachers maintaining their clinical skills.

The nurse teacher interviewees were also shown to believe that they influence students when learning about nursing, but thought students' own peers and clinical staff were a more important influence. Caring for students was seen as desirable by the interviewees but different in terms of the quality and quantity of care they would give to patients. These findings were in direct contrast to that of the student nurse data which showed nurse teachers as being the most frequently mentioned influence when learning about nursing. Nursing for both groups was defined as clinical nursing practice.

Generally the findings of the student nurse data analysis are, however, similar in a number of respects to the findings of analysis of the other data sets. For example, the need for more clinical teaching and clinical practice are identified as important issues. Variations in the findings are that, whilst self–directed study is an important feature of the students' courses, students are not in receipt of teaching likely to develop self–directed learning skills. Also development of problem–solving skills is a further area of deficit. Therefore it can be concluded that not only do the students surveyed feel there is not enough clinical practice or practical skills teaching, but one of the most basic skills of nursing practice, that of problem–solving, is an under–addressed topic in their courses. There is therefore a clear need for nurse educators to address these areas. For example, if a large proportion of students' time is taken up with self–directed learning projects there is an obvious need to equip students with the skills needed for these activities. Also nurse teachers need to be mindful of their facilitative role when students are given self–directed learning tasks. In addition equipping students with the necessary skills for clinical practice is plainly of vital importance. Provision of clinical experiences and practical skills training are further areas which require consideration by nurse curriculum developers.

Student nurse attitudes to nursing care delivery were considered through measurement of PMQX scores. It was found that the student sample generally had high PMQX scores. Females and third year students were shown to have significantly higher scores than the rest of the sample. It was, however, contended that patient–centred attitudes was not an innate attribute but one that could be learnt through effective nurse education programmes. The high PMQX scores gives rise to conclusions that, although there are apparent shortcomings in the courses the students are undertaking, generally the students are developing appropriate attitudes to care delivery.

Indications are also that students in the sample are being treated in ways likely to develop positive self–esteem. For example, the positive responses to statements relating to being treated as an adult, and as an individual, are seen as an indication that the majority of students surveyed are likely to have positive self–esteems. The students are therefore seen to be reasonably cared for by their educators. Care in this context is defined as nurse educators provided effective teaching and learning environments, which will empower and enthuse students, and facilitate students to developing appropriate attitudes and skills necessary for effective patient delivery. Central to this definition, whether it be care for students or care for patients, is in a professional context treating people as individuals, who have their own personal biographies, their own hopes and desires and fears and anxieties, and their own needs and goals in life.

Future areas of research arising out of the results of this study

It was identified at the beginning of this book that the definition of attitude being deployed in the study was that attitudes have cognitive, affective and behavioural components. The cognitive and affective components of attitudes have been explored with regard to the multi–faceted concepts of student–centred learning and teaching and patient–centred care. It is believed that further study is warranted into how these ideas and beliefs are translated into educational and nursing situations. For example, observations of nurse teacher/student nurse interactions would provide evidence of the adoption (or non–adoption) of the ideas and beliefs identified in this book. Similarly observations of student nurses' clinical practice would give verification of how the high PMQX scores findings are related to students' behaviour in clinical practice. Interviews with clinical staff and those acting as students' mentors would give further evidence to how students are seen to approach patient care delivery. Finally patient interviews would not only verify appropriate student–nurse behaviours, but give further insight into what caring attitudes and behaviours are valued by those in receipt of nursing care.

Bibliography

Acton L, Gough P, & McCormack B (1992) 'The clinical nurse teacher debate.' *Nursing Times* 88,32,38–39

Akinsanya J (1987) 'Teaching by contract.' *Senior Nurse* 7,6,26–27

Alderton JS (1983) 'In training – but I want to be educated.' *Nurse Education Today* 3,2, 29–31

Alexander MF (1982) 'Integrating theory and practice in nursing.' *Nursing Times Occasional* Paper, 78, 17

Alexander MF (1984) 'Learning to nurse: Beginning has implications for continuing.' *Nursing Times* 4,1, 4–7

Allcock N (1992) 'Teaching the skills of assessment through the use of an experiential workshop.' *Nurse Education Today* 12,287–292

Anderson LR & Fishbein M (1965) 'Prediction of attitudes from number, strength and evaluative aspects of beliefs about an attitude object.' *Journal of Perspectives in Social Psychology* 2,437–443

Andrews JM (1980) 'The verbal structure of teacher's questions and its impact on class discussions.' *POD Quartley* 3,4,129–163

Arndt MJ (1992) 'Caring as everydayness.' *Journal of Holistic Nursing* 10,4, 285–292

Ashworth P & Morrison P (1991) 'Problems of competence–based nurse education.' *Nurse Education Today* 11,4,256–261

Baillie L (1994) 'Teachers' feelings about participating in clinical practice: An exploratory study.' *Journal of Advanced Nursing* 20,150–159

Baker B (1982) 'First impressions stick.' *Nursing Mirror* 154,24

Baldwin D Hill P & Hanson (1991) 'Performance of psychomotor skills: A comparison of two teaching strategies.' *Journal of Nursing Education* 30,8,367–370

Baly ME (1980) *Nursing and social change* Heinemann, London

Bandura A (1977) 'Self–efficacy: Towards a unifying theory of behaviour change.' *Psychological Review* 84,191–215

Barnett DE (1981) 'Do nurses read? Nurse managers and nursing research reports.' *Nursing Times* 77,50,2131–2134

Barrett–Lennard GT (1962) 'Dimensions of therapist response as causal factors in therapeutic change.' *Psychological Monographs* 76,43

Bauwens EE & Gerhard GG (1987) 'The use of the Watson–Glaser Critical Thinking Appraisal to predict success in a baccalaureate nursing programme.' *Journal of Nursing Education* 26,7,278–281

Baxter RCS (1992) 'Labelling students in nursing.' *Journal of Advanced Nursing* 17,971–974

Beattie A (1987) 'Making a curriculum work'. in Allan P & Jolley M (eds) *The curriculum in nursing education.* Chapman Hall, London

Beckett C & Wall M (1985) 'The role of the clinical facilitator.' *Nurse Education Today* 5, 259–262

Beeman P (1988) 'RN's perceptions of their baccalaureate programmes meeting adult learning needs.' *Journal of Nursing Education* 27, 364–376

Bell J (1984) 'Exposing the hidden curriculum.' *Nursing Mirror* 12, 20–21

Benner P (1984) *From novice to expert..* Addison–Wesley, Menlo Park, California

Benoliel JQ (1984) 'Advancing nursing science, Qualitative approaches.' *Western Journal of Nursing Research* 6,1–8

Betz CL (1985) 'Students in Transition: Imitators of role models.' *Journal of Nursing Education* 24,7,301–303

Bevis EO & Murray JP (1990) 'The essence of the curriculum revolution: Emancipatory teaching.' *Journal of Nursing Education* 29,7,326–331

Bjork IT (1995) 'Neglected conflicts in the discipline of nursing: perceptions of the importance and value of practical skills.' *Journal of Advanced Nursing* 22,6–12

Boreham NC (1977) 'The use of case histories to assess nurses' abilities to solve clinical problems.' *Journal of Advanced Nursing* 2,57–66

Boydell T (1976) 'Experiential learning.' *Manchester Monographs* Manchester

Bradby M (1990) 'Status passage into nursing: Another view of the process of socialization into nursing.' *Journal of Advanced Nursing* 15,10,1220–1225

Bradham CU Dalme FC & Thompson PJ (1990) 'Personality traits valued by practising nurses and measured in nursing students.' *Journal of Nursing Education* 29,5,225–232

Brockett RG (1985) 'Methodological and substantive issues in the measurement of self–directed learning readiness.' *Adult Education Quarterly* 36,1,15–24

Brookes D (1991) 'Self–study programmes and nurse education.' *Nurse Education Today* 11,303–309

Brookes H Emerson T & Saunders M (1983) 'A learner–centred approach.' *Nursing Mirror* June 1st 20–23

Brown GD (1993) 'Accounting for power: Nurse teachers' and students' perceptions of power in their relationships.' *Nurse Education Today* 13,11–120

Brudenell I & Carpenter CS (1990) 'Adult learning styles and attitudes towards computer assisted instruction.' *Journal of Nursing Education* 29,2, 79–83

Bruner J S (1966) *Towards a theory of instruction..* Norton, New York

Bryan J (1991) 'Student–centred learning – facing the challenge'. in Pendleton S & Myles A (eds) *Curriculum planning in nursing education.* Edward Arnold, London

Bryman A & Cramer D (1990) *Quantitative data analysis for social scientists.* Routledge, London
Burber M (1967) *On Judaism.* Shocken Books, New York
Burrell T (1988) *Curriculum design and development.* Prentice Hall, London
Burnard P (1985) 'Future imperfect.' *Senior Nurse* 2,1,8–10
Burnard P (1986a) 'Towards an epistemological basis for experiential learning in nurse education.' *Journal of Advanced Nursing* 12,189–193
Burnard P (1986b) 'Encountering adults.' *Senior Nurse* 4,4, 20–21
Burnard P (1987) 'Teaching the teachers.' *Nursing Times* 83(49,63–65
Burnard P (1988) 'Brainstorming: a practical activity in nurse education.' *Nurse Education Today* 8,354–358
Burnard P (1989a) 'Developing critical ability in nurse education.' *Nurse Education Today* 9,271–275
Burnard P 1989b) 'Playschool.' *Nursing Times* 85,17,36–37
Burnard P (1991) 'The language of experiential learning.' *Journal of Advanced Nursing* 16,873–879
Burnard P (1992a) 'Student nurses' perceptions of experiential learning.' *Nurse Education Today* 12,163–173
Burnard P (1992b) 'Defining experiential learning: nurse tutors' perceptions.' *Nurse Education Today* 12(1) 29–36
Burnard P (1992c) 'Learning from experience: nurse tutors' and student nurses' perceptions of experiential learning in nurse education: some initial findings.' *International Journal of Nursing Studies* 29,2, 151–161
Burnard P (1994) 'Searching for meaning, a method of analysing interview transcriptions with a personal computer.' *Nurse Education Today* 14, 111–117
Burnard P & Chapman C (1990) *Nurse education – the way forward.* Scutari Press, London
Burnard P & Morrison P (1991) 'Client–centred counselling. A study of nurses' attitudes.' *Nurse Education Today* 11,104–109
Burnard P & Morrison P (1992) 'Student's and lecturer's preferred teaching strategies.' *International Journal of Nursing Studies* 29,4,345–353
Byrnes AK (1986) 'Bridging the gap between humanism and behaviourism in nursing education.' *Journal of Nursing Education* 25,7,304–305
Caffrey PA (1994) 'Caring or Codependent'? *Nursing Forum* 29,1,12–17
Cameron BL & Mitchell AM (1993) 'Reflective peer journals: developing authentic nurses.' *Journal of Advanced Nursing* 18,290–297
Cardno J A (1955) 'A notion of attitude.' *Psychology Rep* 1,345–352
Carlisle C (1991) 'The value of contract learning.' *Nursing* 4,26,22–24
Carter SL (1978) 'The nurse educator; Humanist or behaviourist'? *Nursing Outlook* 26,9, 1319–1320
Carter SL (1979) 'The nurse educator.' *Nursing Times* August 2nd 1315–1317
Casey N & Buchan J (1989) 'Recruitment and retention.' *Nursing Standard* 47,3,13–16
Chally PS (1992) 'Empowerment through teaching.' *Journal of Nursing Education* 31,3,117–120

Champion R (1991) 'Devolving responsibility.' *Nursing Times* 87,29
Chandler J (1991) 'Reforming nurse education, implications for teachers and students.' *Nurse Education Today* 11,89–93
Chang AM & Gaskill D (1991) 'Nurses' perceptions of their problem–solving abilities.' *Journal of Advanced Nursing* 16,813–819
Charlesworth G, Kanneh A & Masterson (1992) 'The clinical nurse tutor debate.' *Nursing Times* 88,32
Chiarella EM (1988) 'Ethical dilemmas in curriculum planning.' *Nurse Education Today* 8,96–93
Child D (1986) *Psychology and the teacher.* Holt, Rinehart & Winston, London
Chipman Y (1991) 'Caring its meaning and place in the practice of nursing.' *Journal of Nursing Education* 30,4,171–175
Clark EH & Sleep J (1990) 'The what and how of teaching research.' *Nurse Education Today* 11,172–178
Clarke K (1986) 'Recent developments in self–directed learning.' *Journal of Continuing Education for Nursing*, 17,3,76–80
Clark JAK (1990) 'Self–directed learning skills and clinical performance.' *The University of Southern Mississippi*
Clarke M (1986) 'Action and reflection: practice and theory in nursing.' *Journal of Advanced Nursing* 11,3–11
Clarridge A Couchman WA & Holloway IM (1992) 'Interaction in the classroom, District nurse students and their teachers.' *Nurse Education Today* 12, 200–206
Clifford C (1993) 'The clinical role of the nurse teacher in the UK.' *Journal of Advanced Nursing* 18,281–289
Clinton M (1985) 'Stuck in an educational rut.' *Nursing Mirror* 161,37–38
Cohen JA (1993) 'Caring perspectives in nursing education: liberation, transformation and meaning.' *Journal of Advanced Nursing* 18,621–626
Cohen P (1994) 'Passing the buck'? *Nursing Times* 90,13,28–30
Colman R (1993) 'Patient power.' *Nursing Times* 89,47,50
Condon EH (1992) 'Nursing and the caring metaphor: Gender and political influences on an ethic of care.' *Nursing Outlook* 40,1,14–19
Cook SH (1991) 'Mind the theory:practice gap in nursing.' *Journal of Advanced Nursing* 16,1462–1469
Coombe E, Jabbusch B, Jones M, Pesznecker B, Ruff C & Young K (1981) n incremental approach to self–directed learning.' *Journal of Nursing Education* 20,6, 30–35
Cotanch P (1981) 'Self–actualisation and professional socialisation of nursing students in the clinical laboratory experience.' *Journal of Nursing Education* 20,8,4–18
Cowman S (1993) 'Triangulation: a means of reconciliation in nursing research.' *Journal of Advanced Nursing* 18, 788–792
Craig JL & Page G (1982) 'The questioning skills of nursing instructors.' *Journal of Nursing Education* 21,8,29

Creedy D & Hand B (1994) 'The implementation of problem–based learning: changing the pedagogy in nurse education.' *Journal of Advanced Nursing* 20,696–702
Cronin S & Harrison B (1988) 'Importance of nurse caring behaviours as perceived by patients after myocardial infarction.' .*Heart and Lung* 17,374–380
Crook J (1985) 'A validation study of a self–directed learning readiness scale.' *Journal of Nursing Education* 24,7, 274–279
Crotty M (1993a) 'The emerging role of the British nurse teacher in Project 2000 programmes.' A Delphie study. *Journal of Advanced Nursing* 18,150–157
Crotty M (1993b) 'Clinical role activities of nurse teachers in Project 2000 programmes.' *Journal of Advanced Nursing* 18,460–464
Crout L (1980) 'From a learner's point of view.' *Nursing Mirror* July 3rd 14–16
Darbyshire P (1991) 'The American revolution.' *Nursing Times* 87,6,57–58
Darbyshire P (1993) 'In the hall of mirrors.' *Nursing Times* 89,49, 26–30
Darbyshire P (1994) 'In defence of pedagogy: a critique of the notion of andragogy.' *Nurse Education Today* 13,328–335
D'A Slevin S & Lavery MC (1991) 'Self–directed learning and student supervision.' *Nurse Education Today* 11,368–377
Dawson MS (1994) 'Using locus of control to empower student nurses to be professional.' *Nursing Forum* 29,4,10–15
Davidson A (1992) 'Lifting the mask.' *Nursing Times* 88,32,51
Davies BD (1984) 'Interviews with student nurses about their training.' *Nurse Education Today* 4,2,136–140
Davies E (1993) 'Clinical role modelling: uncovering hidden knowledge.' *Journal of Advanced Nursing* 18,627–636
Davies PS (1991) 'The meaning of change to individuals within a college of nursing.' *Journal of Advanced Nursing* 16,108–115
DeCoux VM (1990) 'Kolb's learning style inventory, a review of its application in nursing research.' *Journal of Nursing Education* 29,5, 202–207
Denzin N (1970) 'Strategies of multiple triangulation'. in *The Research Act.* McGraw Hill, New York
Demirbag BC & Ridenour N (1995) 'Perceptions of learning needs and preferred learning methods about AIDS/HIV amongst registered nurses working in the community in Texas.' *Journal of Continuing Education in Nursing* 26,3,129–134
Dempsey PA & Dempsey AD (1992) *Nursing research with basic statistical applications.* Jones and Bartlett, Boston
Dewey J (1933) 'How we think.' DC Heath, Boston
Diekelmann N (1990) 'Nursing education: Caring, dialogue and practice.' *Journal of Nursing Education* 29,7, 300–305
Diekelmann N (1993) 'Behavioural pedagogy: a heideggerian hermeneutic analysis of the lived experiences of students and teachers in baccalaureate nursing education.' *Journal of Nursing Education* 32,6,245–249
Dingwall R, Rafferty AM & Webster C (1988) *The social history of nursing.* Routledge, London

Di Rienzo JN (1983) 'Before client care – an interactive conference.' *Journal of Nursing Education* 22,2,84–86
Dixon E (1991) 'Nurse readiness and time spent in self–directed learning.' *Journal of Continuing Education in Nursing* 22,5,215–217
Dootson S (1995) 'An indepth study of triangulation.' *Journal of Advanced Nursing* 22,183–187
Dowie S & Park C (1988) 'Relating nursing theory to students' life experiences.' *Nurse Education Today* 8,4,191–196
Dufault MA (1985) 'Changing the locus of control of registered nurse students with a futuristic–orientated course.' *Journal of Nursing Education* 24,8,314–320
Duffy P 1985 'Future imperfect.' *Senior Nurse* 2,1,8–10
Duffy BSC (1986) 'Learning theories and the ward tutorial.' *Nurse Education Today* 6,23–27
Dunlop MJ (1986) 'Is a science of caring possible.' *Journal of Advanced Nursing* 11,661–670
Dux CM (1989) 'An investigation into whether nurse teachers take into account the individual learning styles of their students when formulating teaching strategies.' *Nurse Education Today* 9,3,186–191
Dzurec LC & Abraham IL (1993) 'The nature of inquiry: Linking quantitative and qualitative research.' *Advances in Nursing Science* 16,1,73–79
Eason FR & Corbett RW (1991) 'Effective teacher characteristics identified by adult learners in nursing.' *Journal on Continuing Education in Nursing* 22,1,21–23
Elias JL (1979) 'Andragogy revisited.' *Adult Education* 29,252–256
Elkan R & Robinson J (1995) 'Project 2000: a review of the literature.' *Journal of Advanced Nursing* 22,386–392
Ellis L (1980) 'An investigation of nursing students self–concept levels.' *Nursing Research* 29,6,389–390
Emblen JD & Gray GT (1990) 'Comparison of nurses self–directed learning activities.' *Journal of Continuing Education in Nursing* 21,56–61
English National Board (1989) *Project 2000 A new preparation for practice.* ENB London
English National Board (1993) *Applicant handbook.* ENB, Bristol
English National Board (1993) *Degrees combined with nursing and midwifery qualifications.* ENB, London
Ennis R (1962) 'A concept of critical thinking.' *Harvard Educational Review* 32,1,81–111
Ennis R (1985) 'A logical base for measuring critical thinking skills.' *Educational Leadership* 43,44–48
Fabricius J (1991) 'Learning to work with feelings, psycho dynamic understanding and small group work with junior student nurses.' *Nurse Education Today* 11,134–142
Farabaugh N (1984) 'Do nurse educators promote burnout'? *International Nursing Review* 31,2,47–52
Farmer ES (1992) 'Integrating research and practice.' *Nursing Practice* 5,1,2–7

Farrand LL Holzemer WL & Schleutermam JA (1982) 'A study of construct validity simulations as a measure of nurse practitioners' prblem–solving skills.' *Nursing Research* 31,1,37–42

Fawcett TN & McQueen A (1994) 'Clinical credibility and the role of the nurse teacher.' *Nurse Education Today* 14,264–271

Fell PJ (1989) 'The Keller Plan in nurse education.' *Vocational aspects of education*, XLI, 109,65–68

Fenton MV (1986) 'Development of the scale of humanistic nursing behaviours.' *Nursing Research* 36,2,82–87

Field L (1989) 'An investigation into the structure, validity and reliability of Gugliemino's self–directed learning readiness scale.' *Adult Education Quarterly* 39,3, 125–139

Fieldhouse F (1992) 'Learning to fail.' *Nursing Times* 88,27,40

Flewellyn BJ & Gosnell DJ (1985) 'Comparison of two approaches to hospital orientation for practice efficacy and preferred learning methods of registrated nurses.' *Journal of Continuing Education in Nursing* 16,5,147–152

Fong CM & McCauley GT (1993) 'Monitoring the nursing, teaching and interpersonal effectiveness of clinical instructors.' *Journal of Nursing Education* 32,7,325–327

Fowler P Walker C Warren T & Scott J (1987) 'An unforgettable experience.' *Nursing Times* April 1st 28–29

Freire P (1972) *Pedagogy of the oppressed.* Penguin, Harmondsworth

French P & Cross D (1992) 'An interpersonal–epistemological curriculum model for nurse education.' *Journal of Advanced Nursing* 17,83–89

Frish N (1988) 'Nursing diagnosis: A curriculum model based on the Nanda list.' *Nurse Education* 13,5

Gallego A & Walter P (1991) 'Preparation of health care teachers for the future.' *Nurse Education Today* 11,94–99

Gates RJ (1989) 'Teacher behaviour: A determinant of student self–esteem?' *Nurse Education Today* 9,207–210

Gibbon C (1989) 'Contract learning in a clinical contest; Report of a case study' *Nurse Education Today* 6,264–270

Gibson CH (1991) 'A concept analysis of empowerment.' *Journal of Advanced Nursing* 16,354–361

Givens W (1990) 'Facilitating the cognitive growth of baccalaureate nursing students using writing strategies for thinking and cognitive development.' *Virginia Polytechnic Institute and State University*

Goodall CJ (1985) 'Applying aspects of educational psychology to the practice of nurse teaching.' *Nurse Education Today* 5, 263–266

Gordon S (1991) 'Fear of caring: The feminist paradox.' *American Journal of Nursing* 91,2,44–48

Gott M (1982) 'Theories of learning and the teaching of nursing.' *Nursing Times Occasional Paper* 78,11,41–44

Greenwood J (1993) 'The apparent desensitization of student nurses during their professional socialisation: a cognitive perspective.' *Journal of Advanced Nursing* 18,1471–1479
Griffin AP (1983) 'A philosophical analysis of caring in nursing.' *Journal of Advanced Nursing* 8,289–295
Gross YT Takazawa ES & Rose CL (1987) 'Critical thinking and nursing research.' *Journal of Nursing Education* 26,8,317–323
Hagell EI (1989) 'Nursing knowledge: woman's knowledge. A sociological perceptive.' *Journal of Advanced Nursing* 14,3,226–233
Hallett CE, Williams A, Orr J, Butterworth T & Collister B (1995) 'The implementation of Project 2000 in the community: a new perspective on community nurses' roles.' *Journal of Advanced Nursing* 21,1159–1166
Hamill C (1995) 'The phenomenon of stress as perceived by Project 2000 student nurses: a case study.' *Journal of Advanced Nursing* 21,528–536
Hamm BH & Brodt D (1982) 'Guts: Teaching assertiveness skills by simulation and gaming.' *Nursing Research* 31,4,246–247
Hammer R & Tufts M (1985) 'Nursings' self image – Nurse educators' responsibility.' *Journal of Nursing Education* 24,7,280–284
Hanson M & Patchett T (1986) 'When the tap runs dry.' *Nursing Times* December 31st, 26–28
Happs SJ (1991) 'Problem posing vs problem solving.' *Nurse Education Today* 11,147–152
Hawkett S (1989) 'A model marriage.' *Nursing Times* 85,1,61–62
Henderson V (1966) *The nature of nursing*. Collier–Macmillan, London
Hegge M (1985) 'A model of continuing education through self–directed learning.' *Journal of Continuing Education in Nursing* 16,6,205–213
Henry C & Tuxill AC (1987) 'The concept of person: Introduction to the health professionals' curriculum.' *Journal of Advanced Nursing* 12,245–249
Hilbert GA & Allen LR (1985) 'The effects of social support on educational outcomes.' *Journal of Nursing Education* 24,2,48–52
Hinton C Martin J & Hall J (1992) 'Changing patterns of student nurse recruitment.' *Nursing Times* 88, 22,38–41
Ho E (1991) 'Towards an epistemological basis for andragogy in midwifery education.' *Nurse Education Today* 11,153–156
Hodges SA (1988) 'Individual learning styles of student nurses, their teachers and ward sisters.' *Journal of Advanced Nursing* 13,341–344
Hodges SA (1991) 'An experiment in the development of empathy in student nurses.' *Journal of Advanced Nursing* 16,11,1296–1300
Hogston R (1995) 'Quality nursing care: a qualitative enquiry.' *Journal of Advanced Nursing* 21,116–124
Holden RJ (1991) 'An analysis of caring: Attitudes,contributions and resolutions.' *Journal of Advanced Nursing* 16,893–898
Holloway I & Penson J (1987) 'Nurse education as social control.' *Nurse Education Today* 7,235–241

Holzemer WL (1986) 'The structure of problem–solving in simulations.' *Nursing Research* 35,4,231–235
Hopkins MA (1981) 'An analysis of nurse educator's orientation: Andragogical or pedagogical?' *Dissertation Abstracts International* 44,43a
Houston M & Weatherston L (1986) 'Creating change in midwifery: Integrating theory and practice through practice–based research groups.' *Midwifery* 2,2,65–70
Hurst B (1993) 'Drama class.' *Nursing Times* 89,1, 30–31
Hurst K (1985) 'Traditional versus progressive education; A review of the literature.' *Nurse Education Today* 5,30–36
Iwasiw CL (1987) 'The role of the teacher in self–directed learning.' *Nurse Education Today* 7,5,222–227
Jacka K & Lewin D (1986) 'Numerical measures of integration.' *Journal of Advanced Nursing* 11,6,679–685
Jacono BJ (1993) 'Caring is loving.' *Journal of Advanced Nursing* 18,192–194
James CR & Clarke BA 1994 'Reflective practice in nursing: issues and implications for nurse education.' *Nurse Education Today* 14,82–90
James N (1989) 'Emotional labour: Skill and work in the social regulation of feelings.' *The Sociological Review* 37,1,15–42
Janhonen S (1991) 'Andragogy as a didactic perspective in attitudes of nurse instructors in Finland.' *Nurse Education Today* 11,278–283
Jarvis P & Gibson S (1980) 'Adult learning and adult education.' *Nursing Times* 76,28, 2071–2074
Jarvis P (1986) 'Nurse education and adult education: A question of person.' *Journal of Advanced Nursing* 11,465–469
Jarvis P (1987) 'Lifelong education and its relevance to nursing.' *Nurse Education Today* 7,49–55
Jarvis P (1992a) 'Theory and practice and preparation of teachers of nursing.' *Nurse Education Today* 12,258–265
Jarvis P (1992b) 'Quality in practice, the role of education.' *Nurse Education Today* 12,3–10
Jarvis P (1992c) 'Reflective practice and nursing.' *Nurse Education Today* 12,174–178
Jasper MA (1994) 'A shortened CFP for graduates – the students' experience of student–centred learning.' *Nurse Education Today* 14,238–244
Jewell SE (1994) 'Patient participation: what does it mean for nurses'? *Journal of Advanced Nursing* 19,433–438
Jinks AM (1993) 'A study of attitudes to gender and nursing stereotypes in newly recruited student nurses.' *Nurse Education Today* 13,287–294
Jinks GH (1991) 'Making the most of practical placements what the nurse teacher can do to maximise the benefits for students.' *Nurse Education Today* 11,127–133
Jones M, Miller C & Tomlinson A (1994) *The current teaching provision for individual learning styles of students in pre–registration diploma programmmes in adult nursing.* ENB, London
Jones SA & Brown LN (1991) 'Critical thinking: Impact on nurse education.' *Journal of Advanced Nursing* 16,529–533

Jones WJ (1980) 'Self–directed learning and student selected goals in nurse education.' *Journal of Advanced Nursing* 6,59–69
Joseph D (1985) 'Humanism as a philosophy for nursing.' *Nursing Forum* 12,4,135–138
Kasch CR (1986) 'Towards a theory of nursing action. Skill and competencies in nurse–patient interaction.' *Nursing Research* 35,4,226–230
Keyzer D (1986) 'Using learning contracts to support change in nursing organisations.' *Nurse Education Today* 6,103–108
Kim JO & Mueller CW (1976) *Factor analysis statistical methods and practical issues.* Sage, Beverly Hills
King IM (1971) *Towards a theory for nursing.* John Wiley, New York
King VG & Gerwig NA (1981) *Humanizing nursing education.* Nursing Resources, Wakefield, Massachusetts
Kintgen–Andrews J (1991) 'Critical thinking and nurse education: Perplexities and insights.' *Journal of Nursing Education* 30,4 152–157
Klug C (1989) 'Changes in self–concept during baccalaureate education.' *Nursing Education* 142,7
Knowles MS (1970) *The modern practice of adult education: Andragogy versus pedagogy.* Association Press, Chicago
Knowles MS (1975) *Self–directed learning A guide for learners and teachers.* Follett Publishing Company, Chicago
Knowles MS (1980) *The modern practice of adult education: From andragogy to pedagogy.* Association Press, Chicago
Kolb DA (1976) *The learning style inventory, technical manual.* McBer, Boston
Kolb DA (1984) *Experiential learning.* Prentice Hall, Englewood Cliffs, New Jersey
Komorita N, Dochring K & Hirchert P (1991) 'Perceptions of caring by nurse educators.' *Journal of Nursing Education* 30,1,23–28
Larson P (1984) 'Important nurse caring behaviours perceived by patients with cancer.' *Oncology Nursing Forum* 11,46–50
Larson P (1986) 'Cancer nurses' perceptions of caring.' *Cancer Nursing* 9,2,86–91
Larson P (1987) 'Comparisons of cancer patients' and professional nurses' perceptions of important caring behaviours.' *Heart and Lung* 16,2,187–193
Laschinger HK & Boss NW (1984) 'Learning styles of nursing students and career choices.' *Journal of Advanced Nursing* 9,375–380
Laschinger HK (1986) 'Learning styles of nursing students and environmental press perceptions of two nursing settings.' *Journal of Advanced Nursing* 11,289–294
Lathlean J (1987) 'Who is the new nurse?' *Nursing Times* 83,47,25–27
Lauder W (1994) 'Beyond reflection: practical wisdom and the practical syllogism.' *Nurse Education Today* 14,91–98
Leach R (1988) 'Student nurse selection an experiential approach.' *Nurse Education Today* 8,359–363
Linares AZ (1989) 'A comparative study of learning characteristics of RN and generic students.' *Journal of Nursing Education* 28,8,354–359
Lindop E (1991) 'Individual stress amongst nurses in training: Why some leave, while others stay.' *Nurse Education Today* 11,2,110–121

Lindsay B (1990) 'The gap between theory and practice.' *Nursing Standard* 5,4,34–35
Livneh C (1988) 'Characteristics of lifelong learners in the human services professions.' *Adult Education Quarterly* 38,3,149–159
Loesch T & Foley R (1988) 'Learning preference differences amongst adults in traditional and non–traditional baccalaureate programmes.' *Adult Education Quarterly* 38,4, 224–233
Logue RE (1984) 'Individual learning: The use of guided study units.' *Nurse Education Today* 3,2,109–111
Lopez KA (1983) 'Role modeling interpersonal skills with beginning nursing students. Gestalt techniques.' *Journal of Nursing Education* 22,3,119–122
Lowdermilk DL & Fishel AH (1991) 'Computer simulations as a measure of nursing students' decision–making skills.' *Journal of Nursing Education* 30,1,34–39
MacLeod MLP (1995) 'What does it mean to be well taught? A hermeneutic course evaluation.' *Journal of Nursing Education* 34,5,197–203
Malin N & Teasdale K (1991) 'Caring v empowerment; considerations for nursing practice.' *Journal of Advanced Nursing* 16,657–662
Mallick J (1977) 'Do nurse educators preach what they want practiced?' *Nursing Outlook* 25,4,244–247
Mallik M (1988) 'A caring curriculum.' *Senior Nurse* 8,9/10,9–11
Mander R (1992) 'See how they learn, experience as the basis of practice.' *Nurse Education Today* 12,11–18
Mangold AM (1991) 'Senior nursing students' and professional nurses' perceptions of effective caring behaviours. A comparative study.' *Journal of Nursing Education* 30,3,134–139
May C (1991) 'Affective neutrality and involvement in nurse–patient relationships: Perceptions of appropriate behaviour amongst nurses in acute medical and surgical wards.' *Journal of Advanced Nursing* 16,552–558
Mazhindu GN (1990) 'Contract learning reconsidered: A critical examination for application in nurse education.' *Journal of Advanced Nursing* 15, 101–109
McAdam C Rankin EJ Love B & Patton D (1989) 'Psychomotor skills as self–directed learning: A study of nursing students perceptions.' *Journal of Advanced Nursing* 14,9,788–796
McCaugherty D (1991a) 'The use of a teaching model to promote reflection and the experiential integration of theory and practice in 1st year student nurses. An action research study.' *Journal of Advanced Nursing* 16,5,534,543
McCaugherty D (1991b) 'The theory practice gap in nurse education: Its causes and possible solutions.' *Journal of Advanced Nursing* 16, 1055–1061
McFall T (1995) 'Let's grow up.' *Nursing Times* 91,3,52
McFarlane JK (1976) 'A charter for caring.' *Journal of Advanced Nursing* 1,187–196
McKenzie L (1977) 'The issue of andragogy.' *Adult Education* 27,225–229
McKenzie P (1985) 'Behavioural objectives and an alternative.' *Nurse Education Today* 5,151–158

McKenzie PM (1987) 'Associate degree programmes in Texas: A survey of the instructor's teaching style and the school's licensure examination.' *Dissertation Abstracts International* 49,109,1b
McMillan MA & Dwyer J (1990) 'Facilitating a match between teaching and learning styles.' *Nurse Education Today* 10,3 186–192
Meize–Grochowski R (1984) 'An analysis of the concept of trust.' *Journal of Advanced Nursing* 9,563–572
Melia KM (1984) 'Student nurses' construction of occupational socialisation.' *Sociology of Health and Illness* 6,2,132–151
Merchant J (1989) 'The challenge of experiential methods in nursing education.' *Nurse Education Today* 9,307–313
Merritt SL (1983) 'Learning style preferences of baccalaureate nursing students.' *Nursing Research* 32,6,367–372
Mezirow J (1981) 'A critical theory of adult education and learning.' *Adult Education* 32,1, 3–24
Miers M (1992) 'Adult education.' *Nursing Times* 88,20,42–44
Milgram S (1974) *Obedience to authority.* Harper Row, New York
Miller A (1982) 'Experience in teaching community health nursing.' *Journal of Nursing Education* 21,4,4–11
Miller A (1985) 'The relationship between nursing theory and nursing practice.' *Journal of Advanced Nursing* 10,417–424
Mitchell ES (1986) 'Multiple triangulation: a methodology for nursing science.' *Advances in Nursing Science* 8,3,18–26
Morrison P (1991) 'The caring attitude in nursing practice: A repertory grid study of trained nurses' perceptions.' *Nurse Education Today* 11,3–12
Morrison P (1992) *Professional caring in practice.* Avebury, Aldershot
Morse JM (1991) 'Negotiating commitment and involvement in the nurse–patient relationship.' *Journal of Advanced Nursing* 16,455–468
Morse JM Solberg SM Neander W Bottorff J & Johnson J (1990) 'Concepts of caring and caring as concept.' *Advances in Nursing Science* 13,1,31–40
Mutzebaugh C & Dunn J (1976) he teacher as a 'reinforcement machine' in the teaching and learning process.' *Journal of Nursing Education* 15,5,27–33
Myco F (1980) ursing research information: Are nurse educators and practitioners seeking it out?' *Journal of Advanced Nursing* 5,6,637–646
Myles A (1991) Independent studies and the curriculum in nursing education'. in Pendleton S & Myles A (ed) *Curriculum planning in nurse education* Edward Arnold, London
Neal MT (1989) Room with a view: Uncovering the essence of the student experience in a clinical training setting. Unpublished PhD thesis.' *University of Maryland*
Nelms TP Jones JM & Gray DP (1993) 'Role modelling: A method for teaching caring in nursing education.' *Journal of Nursing Education* 21,1,18–23
Neuman B (1982) *The Neuman System Model.* Appleton–Century–Croft, New York
Newell R (1994) 'Reflection, art,science or pseudo–science?' *Nurse Education Today* 14,79–81

Newsome GG (1983) 'A comparison of the effects of guided design and lecture teaching strategies on the ability of student nurses to solve problems in clinical settings.' *University of Georgia*

Nielsen BB (1992) 'Applying andragogy in nursing continuing education.' *Journal of Continuing Education in Nursing* 23,4,148–151

Nisbet JD & Entwhistle NJ (1974) 'Educational research methods.' *Unibooks*, New York

Norris CM (1979) 'Self care.' *American Journal of Nursing* 79,3,486–489

Norris J (1986) 'Teaching communication skills, effects of two methods of instruction and selected learner characteristics.' *Journal of Nursing Education* 25,3,102–106

Nunnally JC (1978) *Psychometric theory*. McGraw–Hill, New York

Oddi LF (1988) 'Comparison of self–directed learning scores amongst graduate students in nursing, adult education and law.' *Journal of Continuing Education in Nursing* 19,4,178–181

O'Kell SP (1988) 'A study of the relationships between learning style, readiness for self–directed learning and teaching preference of learner nurses in one health district.' *Nurse Education Today* 8,4,197–204

Orem D (1980) '*Nursing: Concepts of practice.*' McGraw Hill, New York

Orr JG (1990) 'Traditional v Project 2000: Something old something new.' *Nurse Education Today* 10,1,58–62

Ostrow CL (1986) 'The interaction of cognitive style, teaching methodology and cumulative GPA in baccalaureate nursing students.' *Journal of Nursing Education* 25,4,148–155

Pardue SF (1979) 'Blocked and integrated content baccalaureate nursing programmes. A comparative study.' *Nursing Research* 28,5,305–311

Pardue SF (1987) 'Decision–making skills and critical thinking ability among associate degree, diploma, baccalaureate and master's prepared nurses.' *Journal of Nursing Education* 26,9,354–361

Parfitt BA (1989) 'A practical approach to creative teaching: an experiment.' *Journal of Advanced Nursing* 14,8,665–677

Partridge R (1983) 'Learning styles: A review of selected models.' *Journal of Nursing Education* 22,6,244–248

Paterson B & Crawford M (1994) 'Caring in nursing education: an analysis.' *Journal of Advanced Nursing* 19,164–173

Pearson A & Vaughan B (1990) *Nursing models for practice.* Heinemann, London

Peate I (1992) 'Under debate.' *Nursing Times* 88,52,49

Pennington DC (1986) *Essential social psychology.* Edward Arnold, London

Peplau HE (1952) *Interpersonal relationships in nursing.* Putnams & Sons, New York

Perry J (1990) 'Why Project 2000?' *Nursing Standard* 4,25,47

Phillips R (1994) 'Providing student support systems in Project 2000 nurse education programmes – the personal tutor role of nurse teachers.' *Nurse Education Today* 14,216–222

Pinkney–Atkinson VJ (1993) 'Nursing education as adult education: A philosophical standpoint.' *Curationis* 6,2,8–10

Polit D & Hungler B (1991) *Nursing research: Principles and methods.* Lippincott, Philadelphia

Poole MH (1982) 'An assessment of critical thinking skills in nursing students.' *University of Houston*

Pratt DD (1988) 'Andragogy as a relational construct.' *Adult Education Quarterly* 38,3–14

Price PJ (1993) 'Parents' perceptions of quality nursing care.' *Advances in Nursing Science* 16,1,33–41

Prociuk JL (1990) 'Self–directed learning and nursing orientation programmes are they compatible?' *Journal of Continuing Education in Nursing* 21,6,252–256

Pugh EJ (1986) 'Dynamics of teaching–learning interaction.' *Nursing Forum* 15,47–58

Pugh J (1986) 'Avoiding stress: Failing to prepare learners adequately for the realities of clinical practice.' *Senior Nurse* 4,5,6–7

Rachal JR & DeCoux V (1992) 'Nurses and adult educational philosophy: Nurses and non–nurses in graduate adult education programmes.' *Journal of Continuing Education in Nursing* 23,6,253–258

Raichura L (1987) 'Learning by doing.' *Nursing Times* April 1st, 59–61

Raudonis BM (1987) 'Adult education: Its implications for baccalaureate nursing education.' *Journal of Nursing Education* 26,4,164–166

Reid B (1993) 'But we're doing it already: exploring a response to the concept of reflective practice.' *Nurse Education Today* 13,305–309

Reynolds WJ & Presly AS (1988) 'A study of empathy in student nurses.' *Nurse Education Today* 8,123–130

Rice CP (1992) 'Strategies and faculty roles for teaching RN students.' *Nurse Educator* 17,11,33–37

Richardson M (1988) 'Innovating andragogy in a basic nursing course: Evaluation of the self–directed independent study contract with basic nursing students.' *Nurse Education Today* 8,315–324

Richardson S (1987) 'Implementing contract learning in a senior nursing practicum.' *Journal of Advanced Nursing* 12,201–206

Riegel KF (1973) 'Dialectic operations, the final period of cognitive growth.' *Human Development* 16, 346–370

Rideout EM (1994) 'Letting go: rationale and strategies for student–centred approaches to clinical teaching.' *Nurse Education Today* 14,146–151

Riseborough R (1993) 'The use of drama in health education.' *Nursing Standard* 7,15–16

Roethlisberger FJ & Dickson WJ (1939) *Management and the worker.*

Rogers BL (1989) 'Concept analysis and the development of nursing knowledge: The evolutionary cycle.' *Journal of Advanced Nursing* 14,330–335

Rogers C (1969) *Freedom to learn.* Charles E Merrill, Columbus, Ohio

Rolfe G (1993a) 'Towards a theory of student–centred nurse education: Overcoming the constraints of a professional curriculum.' *Nurse Education Today* 13, 149–159

Rolfe G (1993b) 'The patient–centred multi–choice questionnaire: Developing an instrument for the measurement of patient–centredness in student nurses.' *Journal of Advanced Nursing* 18,120–126
Roy C (1976) *Introduction to nursing: An adaptation model.* Prentice Hall, New York
Rush KL Ovelett LL & Watson D (1991) 'Faculty development: The essence of curriculum development.' *Nurse Education Today* 11,121–126
Sarton G (1937) *The history of science and the new humanism.* Harvard University Press, Cambridge
Sartre JPI (1977) *Essays in existentialism.* Citadel Press, New Jersey
Savage J (1987) *Nurses, gender and sexuality.* Heinemann, London
Schare BL Dunn SC Clarke HM Soled SW & Gilman BR (1991) 'The effects of interactive video on cognitive achievement and attitudes towards learning.' *Journal of Nursing Education* 30,3,109–113
Schmidt KL & Fisher JC (1993) 'Effective development and utilisation f self–learning modules.' *Journal of Continuing Education in Nursing* 23,2,54–59
Schmieding NJ (1993) 'Nurse empowerment through context, structure and process.' *Journal of Professional Nursing* 9,4,239–245
Schoen DC (1979) 'Life–long learning: How some participants see it.' *Journal of Continuing Education in Nursing* 10,2,3–16
Schon T (1983) *The reflective practitioner.* Free Press, London
Schroeder C & Neil R (1992) 'Focus groups. Humanistic means of evaluating an HIV/AIDS programme based on caring theory.' *Journal of Clinical Nursing* 1,265–274
Schumann LL (1990) 'Attitudes regarding basic nursing programmes.' *Journal of Nurse Education* 29, 2, 71–78
Seed A (1994) 'Patients to people.' *Journal of Advanced Nursing* 19,738–748
Shane D (1983) *Returning to school.* Prentice–Hall, New York
Shaver KG (1986) *Principles of social psychology.* Lawrence Erlbaum Associates, New York
Shaw ME & Wright JM (1977) *Scales for the measurement of attitudes.* McGraw–Hill, New York
Sheahan J (1981) 'A study of the nurse tutors' role.' *Journal of Advanced Nursing* 6,125–135
Sheahan J (1982) 'Educating teachers of nursing: The attitudes of students.' *Journal of Advanced Nursing* 7,69–77
Sheahan J (1991) 'Concepts of the nursing process amongst nurse teachers and clinical nurses.' *Journal of Advanced Nursing* 16,333–342
Sheenan J (1986) 'Aspects of research methodology.' *Nurse Education Today* 193, 203
Shepherd JM & Brooks KL (1991) 'Self–concept amongst senior students in four types of nursing education.' *Nurse Educator* 16,48–9
Siegel H (1980) 'Critical thinking as an educational ideal.' *The Educational Forum* 45,7–23
Simpson I (1979) '*From student to nurse.*' Cambridge University Press, Cambridge

Skelton R (1994) 'Nursing and empowerment: concepts and strategies.' *Journal of Advanced Nursing* 19,415–423

Smith A & Russell J (1991) 'Using critical learning incidents in nurse education.' *Nurse Education Today* 11,284–291

Smith BEG (1992) 'Linking theory and practice in teaching basic nursing skills.' *Journal of Nursing Education* 31,1,16–23

Smith JP (1994) 'Project 2000 assessed: is nurse education a means or an end?' *Journal of Advanced Nursing* 19,411

Smith L (1987) 'Application of nursing models to curriculum.' *Nurse Education Today* 1,109–115

Smith M (1982) 'Simulation gaming and attitude change.' *Journal of Nursing Education* 21,8

Smith P (1991) 'The nursing process: Raising the profile of emotional care in nursing training.' *Journal of Advanced Nursing* 16,74–81

Sparks RK (1982) 'Problem–solving abilities of graduates from associate and baccalaureate degree programmes.' *Journal of Nursing Education* 21,8

Sprengel A & Kelley J (1992) 'The ethics of caring.' *Journal of Holistic Nursing* 10,3,231–239

St Clair C & Brillhart B (1990) 'Rural nurses as self–directed learners; Overcoming obstacles to continuing education.' *Journal of Continuing Education in Nursing* 21,5,219–223

Stevenson M (1986) 'Curriculum development in action.' *Nurse Education Today* 6,263–269

Stevenson PM (1985) 'A research based method of selecting curriculum content.' *Journal of Advanced Nursing* 10,3–13

Stoduski AH & Stafford SM (1982) 'Disseminating nursing research information in the United Kingdom. Abstrasts from the index of nursing research.' *International Journal of Nursing* 19,4,231–236

Stotts NA (1982) 'A study of the effect of placement and level of behavioural objectives in written prose on the intentional and unintentional learning of undergraduate nursing students.' *Journal of Nursing Education* 21,8

Studdy SJ, Nichol MJ & Fox–Hiley A (1994) 'Teaching and learning clinical skills.' *Nurse Education Today* 14,186–193

Sturmey P (1988) 'Writing behavioural objectives: An evaluation of a simple inexpensive method.' *Journal of Advanced Nursing* 13,496–500

Sutcliffe L (1993) 'Leaps of knowledge.' *Nursing Times* 89,42,34–36

Sweeney JF (1986) 'Nurse education: Learner–centred or teacher–centred?' *Nurse Education Today* 6,6,257–262

Sweeney JF (1990) 'The learner–centredness of two registered general nursing and two registered mental health nursing courses as perceived by third–year student nurses.' *Journal of Advanced Nursing* 15,1208–1219

Tanner CA (1990) 'Reflections on the curriculum revolution.' *Journal of Nursing Education* 29,7,295–298

Taylor BJ (1992) 'From helper to human: A reconceptualisation of the nurse as person.' *Journal of Advanced Nursing* 17,1042–1049

Taylor G (1991) 'Assessing nursing students' understanding.' *Senior Nurse* 11,4,30–31

Taylor J (1993) 'Education can never be neutral – teaching for subversion.' *Nurse Education Today* 13,69–72

Theis EC (1988) 'Nursing students' perceptions of unethical teaching behaviour.' *Journal of Nursing Education* 27,3,102–106

Thorne SE & Robinson CA (1988) 'Reciprocal trust in health care relationships.' *Journal of Advanced Nursing* 13,782–789

Tough A (1971) *The adult's learning projects. A fresh approach to theory and practice in adult learning.* Ontario Institute for Studies in Education, Toronto

United Kingdom Central Council for Nursing, Midwifery and Health Visiting (1986) *Project 2000; A new preparation for practice.* UKCC, London

United Kingdom Central Council for Nursing, Midwifery and Health Visiting (1991) *The Report of the Post Registration.* Education and Practice Project, UKCC, London

Vaughan B (1989) 'Two roles, one job.' *Nursing Times* 85,11,52

Vaughan B (1990) 'Caring – a hidden value.' *Nursing Standard* 4,25,26

Vaughan B (1992) 'Exploring the knowledge of nursing practice.' *Journal of Clinical Nursing* 1,161–166

Vaughan JA (1990) 'Student nurse attitudes to teaching/learning methods.' *Journal of Advanced Nursing* 15,925–933

Waltho BT (1986) 'Contract learning – A student's perspective.' *Nursing Standard*

Weatherston LA (1981) 'Bridging the gap: Liaison betweeen nursing education and nursing service.' *Journal of Advanced Nursing* 6,147–152

Webb C (1979) 'The nursing process: A conflict for the nurse teacher?' *Nursing Times* August 2nd, 1318–1319

Webb C (1986) *Feminist practice in women's health.* John Wiley and Sons, London

Webb C (1989) 'Nursing models in the curriculum.' *Nurse Education Today* 299–306

Whittaker AF (1984) 'Use of contract learning.' *Nurse Education Today* 4,2,36–40

Wiley K (1982) 'Effects of a self–directed learning project and preference for structure on self–directed learning readiness of baccalaureate nursing students.' *Journal of Nursing Education* 21,8,21

Wiley K (1983) 'Effects of a self–directed learning project and preference for structure on self–directed learning readiness.' *Nursing Research* 32,3, 181–185

Wilson J (1992) 'Ready for take–off?' *Nursing Times* 88,10,26–28

Wilson–Barnett J (1988) 'Nursing values: exploring the cliches.' *Journal of Advanced Nursing* 13, 790–796

Wilson–Barnett J, Butterworth T, White E, Twinn S, Davies S & Riley L (1995) 'Clinical support and the Project 2000 nursing student: factors influencing this process.' *Journal of Advanced Nursing* 21,1152–1158

Wiseman RF (1994) 'Role model behaviours in the clinical setting.' *Journal of Nursing Education* 33,9,405–409

Woolley N (1990) 'Nursing diagnosis: Exploring the factors which influence the reasoning process.' *Journal of Advanced Nursing* 15,110–117

Wong J (1979) 'The inability to transfer classroom learning to clinical nursing practice. A learning problem and remedial plan.' *Journal of Advanced Nursing* 4,161–168

Wood V & Rubin S (1992) 'Rita Kennedy. A case analysis for decision–making.' *Nurse Education Today* 12,1,19–24

Woodrow P (1993) 'A case for humanism in nurse education.' *Senior Nurse* 13,5,46–50

Woods R & Barrow R (1985) *A introduction to the philosophy of education*. Methuen, London

Wuest J (1991) 'Learning contracts: A vehicle for increasing student involvement in audio teleconferencing.' *Nurse Education Today* 11,185–190

Zahorik J & Brubaker D (1972) *Towards more humanistic instruction*. WC Brown, Iowa

Appendix 1: SAQ survey instrument

I am currently undertaking a research project the subject of which is student–centred learning.

The focus of this survey is pre–registration nurse education programmes. The survey is not covering midwifery, enrolled nurse conversion or courses leading to a second registration. Therefore please do not include these student groups in your answers.

Your help will be most appreciated by answering the following questions.

Respondent details

Would you please answer by ticking the appropriate box(s)

1.	What is your sex?	Male	☐
		Female	☐
2.	What is your age?	20–29yrs	☐
		30–39yrs	☐
		40–49yrs	☐
		over 50yrs	☐
3.	How long have you been qualified as a nurse teacher?	less than 5yrs	☐
		5 - 10yrs	☐
		over 11yrs	☐
		not appropriate	☐

4. What is your current position?

Details of courses run in the institution

Would you please answer by ticking the appropriate box(s)

1. Type/s of pre–registration course/s offered	Degree	☐
	Diploma	☐
	Pre Project 2000	☐
2. Pre–registration courses offered	Adult	☐
	Mental Health	☐
	Mental Handicap	☐
	Child	☐
3. Number of pre–registration common foundation programme intakes per year or pre–project 2000 intakes	One	☐
	Two	☐
	Three	☐
	Four	☐
	Five	☐
	Six	☐
	More than six	☐
4. Current average size of pre–registration common foundation course intakes or pre–project 2000 intakes	under 20	☐
	20–39	☐
	40–59	☐
	60–79	☐
	80–99	☐
	100–119	☐
	over 120	☐

Please only answer the following questions if the pre–registration courses offered in your institution are project 2000 degree or diploma courses.

If the pre–registration courses offered in your institution are also pre–project 2000 courses please also answer question 7.

If the pre–registration courses offered in your institution are only pre–project 2000 courses please go to question 7.

5. Please give the range of
   - pre–registration common foundation taught class size ....

6. Please give the range of branch programme taught class size.

Adult	....
Mental Health	....
Mental Handicap	....
Child	....

7. Please give the range of pre–project 2000 taught class size.

General	....
Mental Health	....
Mental Handicap	....
Child	....

Student–centred learning and teaching questionnaire

There follows a number of statements regarding student–centred learning.

There are no 'right' or 'wrong' answers.

Please try and answer as honestly as you can and give the first spontaneous answer that comes to you.

Try not to give middle, neutral answers except when it is impossible for you to agree or disagree.

Indicate your feeling with a cross on the scale.

	Strongly Agree				Strongly Disagree
1. The principles of teaching adults do not differ from teaching children.	1	2	3	4	5
2. Self–directed learning is an important feature of student–centred learning and teaching methodologies.	1	2	3	4	5
3. Self–directed study skills are not taught in your institution's pre–registration nurse education programme.	1	2	3	4	5

	Strongly Agree				Strongly Disagree
4. Regular account is taken of students' learning styles in teaching sessions in your institution's pre–registration nurse education programme.	1	2	3	4	5
5. Regular account is taken of students' learning preferences in the teaching sessions in your institution's pre–registration nurse education programme.	1	2	3	4	5
6. Contract learning is not used regularly throughout your institution's pre–registration nurse education programme.	1	2	3	4	5
7. Student–centred learning means active learning.	1	2	3	4	5
8. Nurse teachers do not negotiate with students in regard of teaching and learning methods they use in your institution's pre–registration educational programme.	1	2	3	4	5
9. Student nurses are encouraged to reflect on their clinical nursing experiences.	1	2	3	4	5
10. Student–centred learning and teaching does not involve problem–solving activities.	1	2	3	4	5
11. Critical thinking skills are a valued educational outcome of your pre–registration nurse education course.	1	2	3	4	5

Would you be prepared to participate further in this study	Yes	☐
	No	☐

Thank you for spending the time to answer this questionnaire
your help is much appreciated.

An early return of the questionnaire would be helpful. A stamped addressed envelope is enclosed for this purpose.

Annette M Jinks

Appendix 2:
Respondent details, SAQ survey

Biographical details

Sex	Male	24
	Female	52
Age	20–29yrs	0
	30–39yrs	13
	40–49yrs	48
	over 50yrs	15

Number of years qualified as a nurse teacher

	less than 5yrs	5
	5–10yrs	17
	over 10years	53
	not appropriate	1

Current position

	College Principal/Director	3
	Head of School	2
	Vice Principal	2
	Assistant Principal	1
	Academic Registrar	2
	Head of Department/Head of Pre–registration	7
	Course Director/Leader/Coordinator/Manager	16
	Divisional Head	1
	Senior Educational Manager	5
	Principal Lecturer	6
	Senior Lecturer/Assistant Coordinator	16
	Lecturer	13
	Research Coordinator	1
	Curriculum Adviser	1

Institutional details

Level of courses offered

Degree only	14
Degree and Diploma	7
Degree, Diploma & Certificate	7
Diploma only	27
Diploma and Certificate	18
Certificate	3

Branch programmes offered

Adult only	3
Child only	1
Adult & Mental Health	6
Adult & Mental Handicap	1
Adult & Child	1
Adult, Mental Health & Mental Handicap	15
Adult, Mental Health & Child	18
Adult, Mental Health, Mental Handicap & Child	31

Number of student intakes in a year

One	20
Two	49
Three	7

Numbers of students in and intake

under 20	0
20–39	10
40–59	12
60–79	14
80–99	13
100–119	10
over 120	17

Class sizes in common foundation programmes **

Minimum	Maximum	Range	No of Respondents
5	100	95+	1
5	150	145-	1
10	25	15*	2
10	30	15*	4
10	40	30=	2
10	50	40=	3
10	60	50=	3
10	80	70+	1
10	100	90+	1
10	110	100-	2
10	125	115-	3
10	160	150-	1
15	15	0*	1
15	35	20*	2
15	40	25=	2
15	50	35=	2
15	70	55=	3
15	90	75+	2
15	125	110-	1
20	25	5*	2
20	40	10=	2
20	50	30=	2
20	65	35=	1
20	100	80-	1
20	115	95-	2
20	120	100-	1
20	130	110-	1
20	150	130-	2
20	165	145-	1
25	25	0*	1
25	50	25=	2
25	80	55+	1
25	100	75-	1
25	130	105-	2
25	170	145-	2
30	30	0*	2
30	70	40=	1
35	50	15=	1
40	40	0=	1
40	50	10=	1
45	85	40#	1
45	45	0#	1
40	150	110#	1
50	100	50#	1
60	90	30#	1
80	90	10#	1
85	85	0#	1

Question unanswered 3

** Class size taken to the nearest 5

* Class size reported to be regularly 30 and under (n=15)
# Class size reported to be regularly 45 and over (n=7)
= Class size reported to be on occasions 40–79 (n=26)
+ Class Size reported to be on occasions 80–99 (n=6)
– Class size reported to be on occasions over 100 (n=22)

Appendix 3: Nurse teacher interview schedule

Pre–interview check list
1. Record biographical details of the interviewee
2. Ethics – give assurances regarding confidentiality

Schedule
Student–centred learning and teaching
Lead question
1. How would you define student–centred learning?

Subsidiary questions
2. Do you think self–directed learning is an important feature of student–centred learning?
3. Do you think student–centred learning implies active learning?
4. Do you think problem–solving approaches are a feature of student–centred learning?

Lead question
1. What teaching methods do you regularly use when teaching pre–registration student nurses?

Subsidiary questions
2. How you take account of individual learning preferences?
3. Do you do learning style inventories of the students?
4. Are pre–registration students taught study skills?
5. Are reflective skills taught to students?

Lead question
1. Is andragogy the same as student–centredness?

Subsidiary question
2. What do see are the similarities (or differences) between student–centredness and andragogy?

Lead question

1. How much control do you think students have over their learning?

Lead question

1. Do you think behavioural learning theories are appropriate for use in nurse education?

Subsidiary questions

2. How do you use behavioural learning theories in your teaching?

Lead question

1. How can you be sure that the teaching methods you use are effective?

Lead question

1. Are there any barriers to using your preferred teaching methods?

Patient–centred care

Lead questions

1. What do you believe the values of nursing practice should be?
2. What are your views on use of the nursing process?
3. Do you think patients should be involved in planning their own care?

Lead question

1. Do you think there are any shared values of student– centredness and patient–centredness?

Subsidiary question

2. What are the shared values?

Role modelling theory

Lead question

1. Who do think are the most important people for students learning about nursing?

Subsidiary question

2. Do you think nurse teacher are important role models for student?
3. Do you think the clinical teaching activities of nurse teachers are important?

Lead question

1. Do you believe teachers should care for students?

Subsidiary question

2. How might teachers demonstrate caring behaviours?

Appendix 4: Respondent details, nurse teacher interviews

Sex	Male	3
	Female	17
Age	20–29yrs	0
	30–39yrs	11
	40–49yrs	8
	over 50yrs	1
Number of years qualified as a nurse teacher		
	less than 5yrs	5
	5–10yrs	3
	over 10yrs	8
	not appropriate	4
Current position		
	Senior tutor/lecturer	6
	Lecturer	6
	Head of Department	2
	Course director	2
	Adult branch leader	1
	CFP Leader	1
	Community tutor	1
	Unqualified lecturer	1

Nursing practice speciality

Adult nursing	4
Surgical nursing	1
Renal nursing	2
Acute adult	1
Community nursing	2
Orthopaedic nursing	1
Childrens' nursing	2
Theatre nursing	1
Medical nursing	2
Spinal injuries	1
Intensive care	1
None nurse	1
Health visiting	1

Specialist subject teaching *

Nursing theory	7
Surgical nursing	2
Biological sciences	4
Psychology	2
Management studies	3
Social policy	1
Research	3
Communication	1
Community nursing	3
Late life	1
Adult nursing	3
Health studies	1
Childrens' nursing	2

* some respondents identified more than one specialist subject

Level of teaching undertaken

Degree	4
Diploma	16

Appendix 5: Student nurse questionnaire

I am currently undertaking a research project the subject of which is exploration of the relationships between student–centred learning and patient–centred care.

All your answers will be treated in the strictest confidence. Individual or institutional responses will not be identified in any reports of the research findings.

Your help will be most appreciated by answering the following questions

Section one: Respondent details

Would you please answer by ticking the appropriate box(s)

1. What is your sex?	Male	☐
	Female	☐
2. What is your age?	under 20yrs	☐
	20–29yrs	☐
	30–39yrs	☐
	over 40yrs	☐
3. Which branch programme are you going to study?	Adult	☐
	Mental Health	☐
	Mental Handicap	☐
	Child	☐
	Undecided	☐

Section two: Student–centred teaching and learning questions

Would you please comment on the following statements

1. The most important feature of student–centred learning for me is as follows:

2. Self–directed learning is an important feature of my course.

3. I have been taught self–directed learning skills on my course.

4. Active learning is an important feature of my course.

5. Problem–solving skills are taught on my course

6. I prefer the following teaching/learning methods:

7. I am treated as an adult by the majority of people I have come into contact with during my course so far.

8. The most effective way I have learnt about nursing has been as follows:

9. The most influential people for me in learning about nursing have been as follows:

10. I feel valued as an individual by the majority of people I have come into contact with on my course.

Section three: Patient–centredness questions

There follows a number of statements which might be made by patients when talking to you. For each statement five possible replies are given. Please choose what you think would be the most helpful reply that you could make to each statement and circle the letter corresponding to that reply on the answer sheet.

Thank you for your help in completing this questionnaire

Annette M. Jinks

Appendix 6: Respondent details, student nurse questionnaire

		Total	PMQX section only
Female		185	161
Male		39	31
Ages	under 20	41	39
	20 –29	127	108
	30–39	39	31
	over 40	16	13
	unanswered	1	1
Branch programme preferences	Adult	164	146
	Mental Health	24	16
	Mental Handicap	14	10
	Child	16	15
	Undecided	6	5
Type of programme	Degree	67	59
	Diploma	157	133
	Pre–Project 2000	0	0

Total Population 302 n=224 (PMQX section n=192)
Overall response rate 74.17% (PMQX section 63.58%)

For Product Safety Concerns and Information please contact our EU
representative GPSR@taylorandfrancis.com
Taylor & Francis Verlag GmbH, Kaufingerstraße 24, 80331 München, Germany

www.ingramcontent.com/pod-product-compliance
Ingram Content Group UK Ltd.
Pitfield, Milton Keynes, MK11 3LW, UK
UKHW022203190926
475702UK00003B/171

* 9 7 8 1 1 3 8 6 1 2 2 6 6 *